HEALING THE
THYROID
with AYURVEDA

"This much-needed and timely book presents a road map to what every patient wishes for: a body in perfect balance. Our bodies are home to the greatest hormonal symphony ever played. Your thyroid is one of its conductors. Read this book, follow the guidelines, and feel your body play beautiful music, expressed as vibrant mental and physical health."

WILLIAM SEARS, M.D., AUTHOR OF
THE DR. SEARS T5 WELLNESS PLAN

"*Healing the Thyroid with Ayurveda* is a groundbreaking work for humanity's wellness. At this time of massive environmental crises, Marianne's work is necessary for cleansing and healing manifold layers of illness relating to the thyroid and endocrine system. Synthesizing Ayurveda's ancient knowledge with scientific precision, Marianne Teitelbaum puts forth an incisive work, adding another gem to the timeless pantheon of Ayurveda's wisdom."

MAYA TIWARI, VEDIC SCHOLAR, HUMANITARIAN,
AND AUTHOR OF *AYURVEDA: A LIFE OF BALANCE*

"*Healing the Thyroid with Ayurveda* is finally here. Understanding the individual nature of thyroid disease is the only prescription for a cure. Now we can stop treating with blood tests and symptoms and address the source intelligently and Ayurvedically."

JOHN DOUILLARD, D.C., C.A.P., AUTHOR, FORMER
NBA NUTRITIONIST, AND FOUNDER OF LIFESPA.COM

"Dr. Marianne Teitelbaum's new book on thyroid healing offers a completely new and refreshing understanding of thyroid imbalance and the knowledge of how to correct it gently, safely, and fully by addressing root causes unique to each patient. I urge you to read this book and get on the path to healing yourself, your family, and—if you are a doctor—your patients with thyroid conditions. We can only hope that this is the first of many books to come from Dr. Teitelbaum. Read this one now."

NANCY LONSDORF, M.D., AUTHOR OF
THE AGELESS WOMAN AND *A WOMAN'S BEST MEDICINE*

"*Healing the Thyroid with Ayurveda* is a most useful guide to anyone interested in holistic health care. Dr. Marianne Teitelbaum challenges the insufficient modern approaches to treating thyroid dysfunction by pointing to the root causes of the disease and sharing her success with treating it through the methods of a time-tested and science-proven ancient practice. This book is so important! It will intrigue if not revolutionize the way both patients and doctors address disease."

DIVYA ALTER, AUTHOR OF *WHAT TO EAT FOR HOW YOU FEEL*
AND CO-OWNER OF DIVYA'S KITCHEN,
AN AYURVEDIC RESTAURANT IN NEW YORK CITY

"Dr. Marianne Teitelbaum embodies all the wisdom and experience of a great Ayurvedic sage. She explains in language easy enough for the layperson to understand, yet detailed enough for the seasoned practitioner, exactly what we need to do to counteract the alarming epidemic levels of thyroid problems. Going beyond the use of toxic pharmaceuticals and nutraceuticals, Dr. Teitelbaum once and for all gives us a truly natural approach to healing the thyroid gland, sharing her deep knowledge of Ayurvedic herbs, detox recipes, and healing spices. This is a must-read for anyone who is seeking help with their thyroid health. Bravo!"

LISSA COFFEY, AUTHOR OF *SONG DIVINE:*
A NEW LYRICAL RENDITION OF THE BHAGAVAD GITA

"Finally, a book that describes how to treat thyroid disorders without the use of pharmaceuticals or nutraceuticals, using an approach that goes beyond all other thyroid books on the market. If you're seeking natural treatments for your thyroid problems, this is the one book to read this year."

HARI SHARMA, M.D., PHYSICIAN AND
AYURVEDA PRACTITIONER AT WEXNER MEDICAL CENTER,
OHIO STATE UNIVERSITY, AND COAUTHOR OF
AYURVEDIC HEALING AND *CONTEMPORARY AYURVEDA*

"This is the first and most important definitive Ayurvedic contribution on thyroid disease in the West. It is a testimonial to the work of her teacher and mentor, Vaidya Rama Kant Mishra, and his family's lineage of Shaka Vansya Ayurveda."

BILL DEAN, M.D., AUTHOR OF *IC BLADDER PAIN SYNDROME*

HEALING THE
THYROID
with AYURVEDA

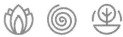

Natural Treatments for Hashimoto's,
Hypothyroidism, and Hyperthyroidism

MARIANNE TEITELBAUM, D.C.

Healing Arts Press
Rochester, Vermont

Healing Arts Press
One Park Street
Rochester, Vermont 05767
www.HealingArtsPress.com

Healing Arts Press is a division of Inner Traditions International

Note to the reader: This book is intended as an informational guide. The remedies, approaches, and techniques described herein are meant to supplement, and not to be a substitute for, professional medical care or treatment. They should not be used to treat a serious ailment without prior consultation with a qualified health care professional.

Library of Congress Cataloging-in-Publication Data
Names: Teitelbaum, Marianne, 1954- author.
Title: Healing the thyroid with ayurveda : natural treatments for Hashimoto's, hypothyroidism, and hyperthyroidism / Marianne Teitelbaum, D.C.
Description: Rochester, Vermont : Healing Arts Press, [2019] | Includes bibliographical references and index.
Identifiers: LCCN 2018028446 (print) | LCCN 2018031672 (ebook) | ISBN 9781620557822 (pbk.) | ISBN 9781620557839 (ebook)
Subjects: LCSH: Thyroid gland—Diseases—Alternative treatment. | Self-care, Health—Popular works.
Classification: LCC RC655 .T45 2019 (print) | LCC RC655 (ebook) | DDC 616.4/4—dc23
LC record available at https://lccn.loc.gov/2018028446

Printed and bound in the United States by McNaughton & Gunn

10   9   8   7   6

Text design by Priscilla H. Baker and layout by Virginia Scott Bowman
This book was typeset in Garamond Premier Pro and Gill Sans with Gentle Sans used as the display typeface.

To send correspondence to the author of this book, mail a first-class letter to the author c/o Inner Traditions • Bear & Company, One Park Street, Rochester, VT 05767, and we will forward the communication, or contact the author directly at **drmteitelbaum.com**.

*I dedicate this book to my mentor and friend,
Vaidya Rama Kant Mishra, who spent countless hours
sitting with me sharing his divine and sacred knowledge,
which continues to infuse and enrich both my life and the
lives of my patients every day. May the work of this
Vedic master, who embodied Ayurveda in its purest form,
continue to echo through the ages.*

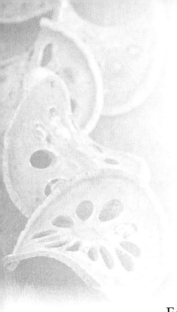

Contents

Foreword

It is truly my good fortune and humble privilege to know and work with an individual such as Dr. Marianne Teitelbaum. She is a bright star, bringing light to the darkness of disease, and bringing to life the true meaning of *healing* and *health*.

As a practicing general endocrinologist, I have found that at least 50 percent of my patients are struggling with autoimmune thyroid disease. Considering the importance of thyroid hormone, which is vital to the proper functioning of virtually every organ, thyroid disease—when not treated adequately—can dramatically affect a person's quality of life. I have often seen that my patients are frustrated by the discordance between their symptoms and the fact that they are being told that their blood work is "normal." What frustrates them more is being prescribed lifelong thyroid medication that they come to realize isn't really helping. We are all born with the intuitive capacity to know when we are out of balance. Patients cannot be satisfied simply because the numbers for their blood work look normal. They want to *feel* normal. They want to *feel* healthy. They want to *feel* the balance of harmony of body, mind, and spirit.

As a health care provider, I am armed with the foundation of a strong medical education, but I strive to not just *treat* patients but also *hear* them. In years past, I found myself searching for something deeper, something more holistic, something that would not just cover or treat the symptoms but get to the seed of the problem. I stumbled on a lecture Dr. Teitelbaum had given in 2014. As someone who also practices meditation and yoga, I was fascinated to hear her call the healthy bacteria living in our digestive system *yoginis,* and to categorize them as a component of the brain of our immune system. She astutely wove together the connections between traditional physiology and the wisdom of Ayurveda, And *it all made sense.* It felt as if I had found the other half of the puzzle. I knew I had to meet her and learn from her, and I did. In fact, I myself went as a patient.

One of our biggest blessings in life is good, balanced health—and it's something that I think we often take for granted. I like to see the body as a sacred shrine—nicely housing our many organs and glands—and a universe of its own. It is truly amazing how the trillions of cells in our body work together tirelessly, in harmony, even when we are sleeping, without our doing anything to make that happen. Our physical body is a tool, an instrument with which we perceive and interact in the world. In its original state of good health, not only does the body function properly, but it has the innate capacity to heal. However, we are living in an age where we push our bodies. We seem to be busier than ever, eating quickly and at the wrong times, sleeping insufficiently and at the wrong times, eating convenient but highly processed foods, and leading a sedentary lifestyle.

These factors, taken together, contribute to a vicious cycle of *dis-ease* in which the body loses its innate quality of being in balance. As a result, we are in the midst of a serious health crisis. Chronic diseases such as diabetes, heart disease, and obesity are increasing at epidemic rates, and they are appearing at a younger age of onset. The incidence of autoimmune thyroid disease, a lesser known but equally devastating disease, is also increasing. There are many theories as to why this is so, and we have yet to determine which among them rings true, but what is readily apparent is that despite the increasing range of synthetic and natural thyroid hormone supplements and medications, patients aren't necessarily feeling better, despite their blood work seeming to be improved.

Ayurveda is a system of medicine dating back thousands of years and rooted in India. *Ayur* means "life" and *veda* means "science"; in other words, Ayurveda is the science of life. According to Ayurveda, our natural state is balance and health, and any symptom or disease is a manifestation of a deviation from our natural state. The beauty of this perspective is that it allows us to detect a state of imbalance—that is, the root of disease—before it grows serious enough to appear in our blood work. It recognizes and values the body's original state of balance as the primary defense against disease.

When I went to see Dr. Teitelbaum as a patient, she spoke with me for a while, inquiring after my state of physical and emotional health, and then she went into a profound healing silence as she analyzed my pulse. From this one energetic and sensate diagnostic, she was able to tell the story of my inner physical world with extreme accuracy, far beyond what traditional blood work had suggested.

From a thyroid perspective, allopathic medicine treats the symptoms of the imbalance. Ayurveda focuses on the root—that is, *why did we develop the imbalance?* Through her years of experience and innate understanding of the body and Ayurvedic principles, Dr. Teitelbaum has successfully treated many patients with thyroid problems. I have entrusted many of my own patients to her care. Many of them had been struggling for decades, treating thyroid disease only on the surface. By healing these patients from the ground up—focusing at the root— Dr. Teitelbaum was able to systematically and successfully restore the thyroid gland to health.

So, dear readers, I have one pure wish for each of you: Thyroid disease can have a devastating and grueling effect on our daily functioning and quality of life. As you read this book and take in Dr. Teitelbaum's expertise in bringing the thyroid back to balance, may your journey be one of transformation, upliftment, and healing.

I sincerely thank and commend Dr. Teitelbaum for her utmost dedication, her humility, and her wisdom. Her mission is to serve and heal. In a world where pharmaceuticals are omnipresent, she has demonstrated inspiring courage in reawakening the ancient science of

Ayurveda and recognizing its true value. She is a real pioneer in taking true healing back to its roots and restoring us to harmony and health. For that, we should all be grateful.

NAMASTE AND OM SHANTI,
ANJALI GROVER, M.D.

Dr. Anjali Grover is an endocrinologist specializing in the treatment of diabetes, thyroid disorders, and other hormonal disorders and deficiencies. She holds a B.A. in economics from Barnard College/Columbia University and an M.D. from Stony Brook University Medical Center. Dr. Grover completed her internal medicine residency at NYU Langone Medical Center and her fellowship training at Brigham and Women's Hospital and Harvard Medical School. She worked as a clinical endocrinologist at NYU Medical Center for a number of years and is now currently working at Hackensack Meridian *Health* Mountainside Medical Group. She loves building relationships with her patients and striving to incorporate meditation practices into health and healing.

Acknowledgments

Writing this book has been deeply rewarding, reinforcing my love of Ayurveda and all of the people who have brought meaning to my life, starting with my loving and nurturing parents, who always supported everything I wanted to do. I wish with all my heart that they could be here to celebrate the publication of my book. My children, Eric and Carly, are the joys of my life—and reliable consultants when technology fails me or I fail it. My husband, Larry, is not only my best friend but a shrewd reader who employed his years of editorial experience to refine my manuscript. Of course, I owe thanks to many others for the inspiration and completion of this book. I want to thank my colleagues and patients who prodded me to share my knowledge in a book, as well as my office assistants, Ann Keys and Barb Haslam, both of whom have unfailingly, and for many years, answered the phones ringing off the hook, unpacked one carton after another of herbs, and generally kept my practice running without a hitch. I also want to thank my agent, Anne Marie O'Farrell, who expertly guided me through the publication process, which was a mystery to me, and my publisher, Inner Traditions. This is my first book, and I really couldn't be happier with my collaboration, which has been marked by professionalism and courtesy. I sincerely hope the book will prove instructive to readers as they continue their journey back to radiant and enduring health.

Preface

In the early 1960s, a time of great ferment, physicist-philosopher Thomas Kuhn authored an influential book called *The Structure of Scientific Revolutions*. The book rippled through the scientific community, creating waves and opposition as it went. In it, he argued that progress does not always proceed in a straight line but is, rather, subject to periodic paradigm shifts that challenge conventional wisdom. We are in such a moment now.

It is a time of twists and turns. In the years since Kuhn's book, many patients have awoken to the gaps and problems of modern medicine. After all, when the third leading cause of death in the United States is a hospital stay, it is time for some soul-searching—and a concerted effort to avoid hospitalization! Westernized, fast-track versions of holistic medicine came along with new and improved models based on purported "natural" treatments. But these often fell short, offering a facsimile of modern medicine that quite often substituted synthetic vitamins and minerals for pharmaceuticals, while at times maintaining the laser focus on treatment of symptoms. Indeed, the time is ripe for a reassessment of the old models.

Enter The New Ayurveda.

Ironically, it turns out that today the new paradigm Kuhn trumpeted comports with the ancient practice of Indian herbal medicine. The New Ayurveda draws on eternal principles to treat the underlying cause(s) of illness. It takes into account our modern ills and develops a series of new protocols, and it delivers on the promise of personalized medicine that we have been hearing so much about.

Let's take a look at the pitfalls of modern and purported holistic medicine through the eyes of two of my patients.

Elizabeth and Megan, twins, born thirteen years ago, were happily brought into this world to two adoring parents. Their parents followed all of their pediatrician's advice to ensure a healthy life for their beautiful girls. However, after a round of immunizations at age two, the parents noticed, much to their dismay, that the girls had locks of hair falling out in clumps. At first they brushed it off, hoping it would stop on its own, but as the weeks went by, the girls eventually lost all of their hair, including their eyebrows and bodily hair.

Frantic, the parents rushed the twins to their pediatrician, who, after his examination, referred them to Children's Hospital. Doctors there determined that the girls had inherited their mother's hypothyroid condition, which explained the hair loss. The girls were immediately placed on a thyroid hormone and began a torturous round of steroid injections into their scalps, leaving them forever fearful of doctors and, worse, still bald.

Their doctors encouraged the parents to bring their children to a support group, which met once a year in different parts of the country, so that the girls would grow up knowing that there were others who were suffering a similar fate. At one of these meetings they heard about a renowned holistic practitioner who performed extensive blood work and as a matter of course prescribed numerous nutraceuticals for thyroid patients, including multivitamins, minerals, L-glutamine, glutathione, turmeric, vitamin D, coenzymes, alpha-lipoic acid, ashwagandha, and vitamin B complex. They made an appointment with the practitioner, and after their initial consultation, it was decided that they would keep the girls on their thyroid hormone as they followed their new supplement program. Excited and hopeful at first, the family became discouraged and disillusioned over the next two years when nothing changed and the girls felt nauseous from taking their daily deluge of pills. That's when the family found its way to my Ayurvedic practice.

Having treated many thousands of thyroid cases, I knew that their medical doctors had taken the wrong approach by focusing solely on the thyroid gland's insufficiency and doing nothing to correct the immune system's assault on the gland. I also knew that the thyroid hormone they had prescribed to the girls was doing more harm than good—by giving the hormone, they were unwittingly shutting down the girls' need to make their own supply of hormone.

The naturopath at least tried to fix their immune systems, but his mistake was that he prescribed some synthetic nutraceuticals, which, like pharmaceuticals, can cause numerous side effects. The other problem with the protocol he prescribed was that it contained too many tablets to be taken orally, without any attention focused on the liver, which would have to process all these remedies, disturbing its function and thus creating an even stronger autoimmune response (much more on this later).

Since pharmaceutical medication is outside the scope of my practice, I told the parents that it was up to them to decide if they wanted to lower the dosage of the girls' thyroid hormone as they began the Ayurvedic protocol I designed for them. Through the next several weeks and months the dosage was tapered and eventually discontinued as we shifted our emphasis to fixing the reasons their immune system was strained to the point that it was actually attacking their thyroid gland, making it impossible for the gland to work, causing their baldness.

Our approach was to use truly natural remedies consisting of herbs, food, and spices to bring the immune system back on track, allowing it to stop its incessant attacks on the thyroid gland. Then we added support for the gland itself to help it heal on its own, without relying on the hormone. In addition, every effort was made to keep the oral medications to a minimum, using other delivery systems of the herbs (via transdermal application, homeopathic dilutions of the herbs given in water to be slowly sipped all day, as well as the use of very dilute teas) in order to keep the load off the liver.

Slowly but surely little patches of hair began to grow, month after month, until both regained their full head of lustrous brown hair—which they had also inherited from their mother. In addition, with health and balance restored to their immune system, which had been disrupted by too many immunizations at one time, they were relieved of their sensitivities to gluten, dairy, and other foods. Better yet, the parents knew that addressing all of these problems at a young age would help protect the girls against developing other autoimmune diseases, such as fibromyalgia and lupus, later in life.

It is for Elizabeth and Megan and the thousands of patients in similar straits that I write this book.

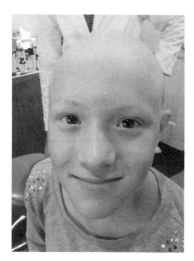 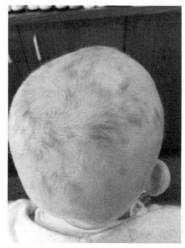

Elizabeth at her third-month checkup

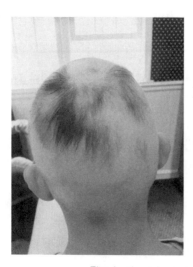 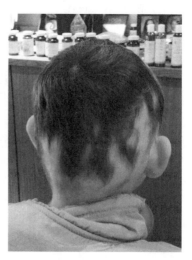

Elizabeth at her sixth-month checkup

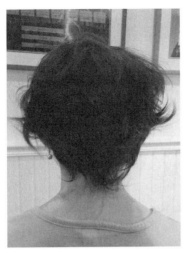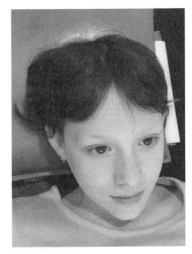

Elizabeth at her one-year checkup

What we know is that America is reeling from an epidemic of ill health that drives people to despair and to doctors. The litany is familiar: cancer, heart disease, autoimmune diseases, and digestive disturbances, with the latter two often one and the same. How can we be so sick in one of the most technologically advanced countries in the world, home to superior diagnostic equipment, wonder drugs, and esteemed medical institutions? We are at a point where both allopathic and holistic medicine need the kind of paradigm shift suggested by Kuhn, whether in the treatment of thyroid disease or in any number of other diseases.

Allopathic doctors are trained to look for and treat disease with a range of side effect–laden pharmaceuticals that only address symptoms and upset our body ecologies. Through no fault of their own, they have no method to detect underlying imbalances early on, before disease sets in, when they are much easier to manage.

Holistic medicine is in its infancy in the United States, and as with any new discipline, there is a great deal of experimentation. Inevitably and understandably, mistakes are made. Holistic practitioners are on the right track with their use of natural alternatives to pharmaceutical medicines. But herein lies the problem: in addition to using various herbs and foods for healing, many also incorporate the use of numerous synthetic vitamins, minerals, amino acids, and so forth. Upon closer inspection, these so-called natural products, often placed under the category of nutraceuticals, are nearly as problematic as drugs, made as they are in a lab and divorced from nature. Like pharmaceuticals, they have an effect, but at what cost? While these remedies may decrease some symptoms, all too often patients become sick over time from taking this man-made version of vitamins in much higher doses than naturally occur in food. The body recognizes these synthetic supplements as toxins, which makes the kidneys and liver work overtime to rid the body of these chemicals. Thus, if we are going to present a truly *natural* alternative to allopathic medicine, then the treatment needs to consist of remedies that are grown in *nature.*

Not only that, we have to consider the strain on the liver from swallowing so many supplements, even if some of them are herbal and truly natural. It is the job of the liver to process everything we swallow, so we don't want to overwhelm it with so many tablets and concoctions. "How much can the liver take?" I remember hearing over and over again as Vaidya Mishra and I would examine patients who would present to us a long laundry list of supplements (both synthetic and natural) they were taking.

This book will present to you a truly alternative, alternative medicine: Ayurveda.

Ayurveda is a 5,000-year-old traditional system of Indian herbal medicine. Well before Hippocrates, ancient Indian seers developed a comprehensive system of healing that addressed imbalances and the root causes of those imbalances, with the ideal goal of preventing illness when possible and reversing it when not.

A chiropractor by training, I became interested in Ayurveda some thirty years ago when I decided to study herbs in an effort to help my patients overcome intractable health problems. In short order I discovered that American indigenous herbs were lying fallow in the fields, undiscovered and unknown to the masses. The United States, a young country, never had the opportunity to develop a full-scale herbal pharmacopoeia. As a result, there were few herbal experts with whom to study.

I went on to study with various nutritionists around the country and learned how to use nutraceuticals, conducting a trial run of that approach in the early years of my practice, and suffering deep setbacks along with my patients. More determined than ever, I turned to Ayurveda, which I had heard of through my exposure to meditation and Eastern culture. With this modality, I found a glimmer of success—my patients started to get better. But the seminal moment came in 1999. That year, I was introduced to and started studying with Vaidya Rama Kant Mishra, who had come to America from India to develop Ayurvedic formulas for the premier Ayurvedic herbal company in the United States.

Dr. Mishra held an exalted place in the Ayurvedic pantheon, having descended from a line of "Raj Vaidyas," or Ayurvedic doctors who held the distinction of being chosen to treat the royalty of India. And now he was training me! Over the next seventeen years Dr. Mishra sat by my side as we saw hundreds of patients, painstakingly teaching me how to use five hundred herbal formulas to treat every conceivable disease and condition.

But he did so much more. My office became his laboratory, so to speak. Dr. Mishra soon discovered that American patients were unable to metabolize many of the herbs he used in India, could not tolerate the cleansing techniques recommended in the ancient texts, and suffered from different modern maladies not discussed in the ancient texts, such as fibromyalgia and many others. In addition, many presented with very delicate physiologies resulting from the overuse of pharmaceuticals and the ingestion of processed foods. So in concert with me, Dr. Mishra adapted and reoriented the traditional practice into what we today call The New Ayurveda, combining the wisdom of the seers with modern research.

Compared to traditional practice, The New Ayurveda incorporates a few of Dr. Mishra's key innovations:

His remedies call for just a pinch or two of herbs in a quart of boiled water instead of the typical one teaspoon per cup of boiled water. Everything we swallow passes through the liver; however, the American liver tends to be so overwhelmed by excesses of pharmaceuticals, nutraceuticals, and processed foods that in many cases it does not tolerate normal doses of the herbs.

He introduced the use of herbal transdermal creams, where herbs are taken directly into the blood from the skin, thus bypassing the liver, giving it a much-needed break.

A special process was also developed by Dr. Mishra whereby the pranic energy of the herb is extracted, filtering out the crude physical herb and infusing just the vibration or intelligence of the herb into organic yellow squash syrup. Because these resultant nectar glyceride drops contain none of the physical molecules of the herb, there is no crude herb for the hot reactive liver to attack and oxidize. Yet at the same time the cellular system, organs, and glands can enjoy the exact same benefits as if the physical herb were present. Keep in mind it is the pranic energy that produces the effects on the physiology. Thus, by incorporating this ingenious delivery system, numerous herbs can be given by drops taken in a liter of water and sipped slowly throughout the day, preventing the extreme stress to the liver that comes from swallowing herbs, vitamins, minerals, amino acids, enzymes, pharmaceuticals, and so forth.

Daily oil massage—a common Ayurvedic practice to remove toxins, lubricate the joints, and slow down the aging process—was revised by Dr. Mishra. In The New Ayurveda, traditional sesame oil is replaced with olive or almond oil in the colder months for people with light skin. We found that lighter-skinned patients could not handle the heavier sesame oil used on Indian patients—the oils sat on their skin, not absorbing, and created too much heat on the body, since sesame oil is considered a heating oil. We also recommend the use of coconut oil in the summer months, regardless of whether they have light or dark skin, as coconut oil, a cool oil, can pacify the effects of heat on our bodies as it accumulates throughout the summer months.

Cleansing techniques recommended in the ancient texts were updated to accommodate the modern toxins that those long-ago doctors couldn't have foreseen: pesticides, pharmaceuticals, nutraceuticals, and air pollution, for example.

The ancient doctors provided us with the textbooks of Ayurveda to teach future doctors how to treat a wide variety of ailments. They did say this, however: they would leave the textbooks open for the future doctors to add new chapters to their books, because they could not possibly foresee what would happen in the future. And this is precisely what Vaidya Mishra did as we saw patients together. These changes presented above represent the upgrades he made, keeping Ayurveda relevant and effective in this modern era.

Once we overcame the various hurdles we encountered in the early years, hundreds and hundreds of patients came to our office, streaming in from all around the world, and slowly regained their health. We reported our findings to numerous Ayurvedic associations and clinics around the country. Our reputations grew as word spread about the work we were doing. After lectures, people would invariably run up to me and ask me to write a book, so I have dedicated myself to compiling all the knowledge I gained from my mentor in order to share it with patients like Elizabeth and Megan, and with doctors who wish to adopt these protocols.

I focus on the thyroid for good reason. I have seen more than ninety thousand patients presenting with every conceivable illness over the last thirty years of my practice. But by far I treat more people with thyroid conditions than anything else. In a typical day, at least half of my patients have some form of thyroid malfunction. The stressors of modern life can weaken the thyroid gland, with consequences for the entire physiology that can result in a wide range of confounding chronic maladies.

The ancients who wrote the textbooks on Ayurveda warned doctors, "If all you do is give herbs to the patient, you are a bad doctor." They went on to say that in order to effectively treat patients, you must first and foremost diagnose the underlying *hetu*, as they called it, referring to the underlying cause of the problem, or the *etiology*, as it is called today. Next you must teach patients proper diet, daily routine, and cleansing techniques in order to effect true and lasting changes in their health.

There are numerous reasons that someone might develop a thyroid problem, and those reasons will vary depending on the patient. Through pulse diagnosis and pertinent questions, you can discover the root causes, address them, and *then* support the thyroid. Without getting to the root of the problem, treatment of the thyroid is destined to provide minimal, if any, results.

One thing that I have learned in these past thirty years is that whatever the manifestation of disease, it is just a symptom of some underlying problem that needs to be addressed. Cancer? A symptom—what caused it? Rheumatoid arthritis? A symptom—dig deeper to find the etiology. Hashimoto's disease? Why is the immune system misfiring and attacking the thyroid? Fix that, and you can watch the thyroid perk up.

When underlying causes are addressed, the patient will have great success in overcoming an ailment and regaining balanced health. Above all, we must resist the temptation to treat only the obvious; the cause is usually far removed from the symptom. That is the credo of this book. It is a simple message, yet it is often overlooked as the medical community strives to help their patients regain their health.

I write this book secure in the knowledge that the ancient art of Ayurveda is the medicine of the future. In recent years, the World Health Organization (WHO) has recognized the efficacy of Ayurveda and encouraged further research and study, noting its upsurge in the West. WHO forecasts a $5 trillion market for herbs worldwide by 2050.

An article in the *Journal of Ayurveda and Integrative Medicine* summed it up: "If [Ayurveda] opens up to incorporate emerging new knowledge into mainstream Ayurveda while maintaining fidelity to Ayurvedic fundamentals, it will certainly provide a broad-based opportunity to address the majority of problems that have emerged from the advent of new diseases and healthcare related issues."

That is a challenge I readily accept.

INTRODUCTION
Traditional Healing for a New Age

Thyroid problems are at an all-time high. More than 12 percent of the U.S. population will develop a thyroid condition during their lifetime. That equates to an estimated 20 million Americans with some form of thyroid disease, with up to 60 percent of them unaware of their condition. Hashimoto's thyroiditis affects 14 million people in the United States alone, making it not only the most common form of thyroiditis but also the most common autoimmune disease in America. This highly vulnerable gland is extremely sensitive to any and all stressors: radiation, chemicals, infections, and mental, emotional, and physical stress. Is it any wonder that thyroid problems are skyrocketing?

Americans love to learn all they can about their health problems, incessantly reading about each and every disease on the internet, looking for anything that can alleviate their symptoms. The problem is that people are searching for advice in a country with no genuine tradition of holistic healing.

Ayurveda is the most ancient and yet fastest-growing traditional health care system in the world, especially in the United States, where we thirst for more natural ways of healing. Our modern allopathic doctors and many holistic practitioners would be wise to explore what these ancient healers had to say about health and adapt it to complement, enrich, and expand our otherwise incomplete health care systems. And that is what I aim to do with this book: discuss the most up-to-date information and research on thyroid malfunction while at the same time showing you how to manage these problems using time-tested methods explained in great detail thousands of years ago.

You will first learn the fundamentals of Ayurveda, which will give you perspective as you subsequently read about the function of the thyroid gland and the numerous factors that affect normal thyroid activity. We will investigate two opposing perspectives on the development of thyroid malfunction. One discussion, based on ancient Ayurvedic wisdom, will rarely mention the thyroid gland, focusing more on the underlying influences that create the thyroid problem in the first place. The thyroid gland is seen more as a victim of these underlying disturbances. The second more modern and perhaps somewhat superficial way of explaining a thyroid condition is to view the problem as just that: a problem with the thyroid gland, ignoring the forces that constantly tug at this beleaguered gland, preventing it from functioning normally.

Let me explain. The ancients talked about principles in nature that govern all the functions of our body. Disruption of these basic governing factors, if not addressed early on, can blossom into full-blown disease. These principles were given the names *vata, pitta,* and *kapha.*

Vata is described as the element of space and air, embodying the qualities of quickness, lightness, dryness, roughness, and movement. Pitta is seen as the fiery element, transforming or "burning up" our food after ingestion. It is also seen as the element that digests and transforms our thoughts and emotions. Kapha, the final element, represents earth and water. This heavier element lubricates the body—the brain and spinal cord, the joints, and the stomach—protecting these areas from the burning of pitta and the drying effects of vata. Due to its unctuous nature, it makes for slow and stable digestion and amiable and relaxed personalities. Kapha can balance excess vata or pitta, calming the effects of the quickness or hyperactivity of vata and soothing the effects of hyperacidity in the body as pitta spirals out of control.

As you read and absorb the concepts in this book and come to understand how the thyroid works or malfunctions—and in the latter case, what to do about it—you will always be drawn back to the deeper knowledge presented in the ancient texts. You will constantly be reminded that while, yes, there is a problem with the thyroid gland, the real and deeper issue is that the elements of vata, pitta, and kapha have been allowed to become imbalanced and wreak havoc in the body. Until you learn to correct these imbalances, you will continue to be prone to and frustrated by thyroid problems, which are, in truth, only symptomatic of a much larger picture.

Ayurveda laid the foundations for modern medicine. The early doctors formulated the various disciplines of medicine and described the first surgical techniques. That knowledge spread from the Vedic culture to Indonesia, infiltrating the healing traditions of Tibet, Sri Lanka, Burma, and other Buddhist countries influenced by Chinese medicine. Eventually the ancient Greeks borrowed this philosophy, renaming vata, pitta, and kapha as air, bile, and phlegm, respectively. Western medical schools followed suit, continuing to emphasize the importance of balance in the body until they began to lose touch with this idea. By the end of the 1800s, health care began to focus more on the symptoms created by malfunction of these three "humors," as they were called, compartmentalizing the body into systems of organs and glands and associated disease states. The focus shifted even more as pharmaceuticals were developed to the point where modern medicine today focuses exclusively on the diagnosis and treatment of disease and which pharmaceuticals to take to suppress the symptoms of that particular disease.

The focus of this book is to bring you back to the dawn of the creation of medicine, back to a time when the body was viewed as a whole, not compartmentalized for the study of disease. We will discuss the thyroid conditions from the often-missed subclinical hypothyroidism to diagnosable hypothyroidism and autoimmune Hashimoto's disease, which are the most common thyroid problems, always with an eye toward the deeper understanding of what causes these problems in the first place. Once we have evaluated the various reasons the thyroid gland malfunctions, then we can turn our thoughts to how to fix them, learning Ayurvedic dietary guidelines, correct daily routine and cleansing protocols, and herbal treatments. We will conclude with herbal remedies for all the maladies that can be caused by a weak thyroid gland, including depression, weight gain, hair loss, constipation, high cholesterol, brain fog, insomnia, heartbeat arrhythmias, low progesterone, heavy and midcycle menstrual bleeding, and more.

Our country lacks a thorough understanding of traditional healing. We never received guidance from wise ancestors to show us how to use our hundreds of herbs for healing. We never developed a firm grasp of what constitutes a good diet and instead developed a taste for highly processed and nutritionally insufficient food. No one ever instructed us on how to rid our bodies of impurities, how to identify imbalances, or how to cultivate our energetic connections with the world in order to remain in harmony physically, mentally, and spiritually. All these issues will be addressed so you come away with a thorough understanding of how to take care of yourself and your family.

If you are like the countless patients I have seen through the years, you are almost totally in the dark regarding your health, caught in the morass of, among other things, conflicting dietary advice: someone recommends you eat just meat and vegetables, someone else suggests you adopt a vegan diet, and yet another voice counsels raw foods only, or perhaps you should go Paleo or low-FODMAP or gluten-, dairy-, or soy-free. What's left to eat? You read about various cleanses and think that they sound harsh, if not outlandish, and come away feeling that they might not be right for you—for good reason! You hear about the latest fads as they come and go, and you wonder, if they were so good, why did they go?

Most of us are bewildered by or skeptical of all the conflicting health advice that is available today, while at the same time feeling that, somewhere deep inside, there must be some unifying truth, some universal principles that teach us how to attain and maintain optimum health. If that description applies to you, then the upcoming pages may bring a sense of relief as you become steeped in sound knowledge that prides itself on getting to the root of the problem without relying on fads that fade as new research is published.

In my experience, if you educate patients about how their bodies work and why they got sick in the first place, they will develop a better understanding of their treatment protocols and, in the end, have a clear idea of what they are trying to accomplish and how to achieve a good outcome. My aim in this book is to help you, the reader, trace the origins of your illness. For this work to be successful, you must relinquish preconceived notions about your health. Keep a perspective on your condition—yes, you have full-blown thyroid symptoms, but *why?* And what can you do about it? You must understand that taking care of your thyroid gland involves more than popping a pill, whether that pill is a prescription medication, a nutraceutical, or an Ayurvedic herb. Proper health care is holistic, encompassing a range of remedies, healing techniques, and healthful lifestyle practices, and it focuses on, above all, balance and harmony. In many respects, health is an ever-evolving mosaic. This book can help you figure out how to make your body work in harmony again, always with an eye toward the deeper principles that caused the disease.

Finally, be reassured: the information is basic, easy to understand and apply. One thing I have heard over and over again from my patients is that the New Ayurveda approach makes sense. It is sound, and it is solid. And though the knowledge comes from India, it doesn't mean that you have to adopt an Indian diet or superimpose Hindu religious rituals on top of your own spiritual values. The information contained in Ayurveda is true for all cultures and all peoples for all times.

The ancient seers said that the timeless knowledge of Ayurveda is present and vibrating in all the cells of our bodies. It is inherent and already known. As you read this book, you will find yourself saying, "Yes, I already knew that at some deep level." And that is what my patients tell me: they had held the keys to radiant health all the time; they only needed someone to show them how to unlock the door. So let's now see how to apply this ancient science to your own health, with particular emphasis on the thyroid gland.

I

What Is Ayurveda?

Nature itself is the best physician.

HIPPOCRATES

The first holistic health conference in America opened to great fanfare in 1975. As with so many innovations, it occurred in California. It brought together 150 of the greatest minds in the emerging field, sparking a spate of holistic health organizations. Here, finally, was a recognition of alternative medicine, an implicit challenge to the medical orthodoxy that had taken root in Western civilization.

Only problem? It was thousands of years late. On the other side of the world, in India, seers held their own gatherings as early as 3000 BCE, producing an elegant system of health care that emphasized prevention, aimed to address the underlying causes of disease, and offered supporting texts with precise protocols that were both prescient and relevant.

In those days, no one talked much about "holistic" medicine because there was no such thing. All medicine was inherently holistic, and none of it was considered "alternative"; it was just medicine.

Just think about it. Ayurveda predates Jesus and Buddha. It is the product of enlightened seers living in an agrarian society who intuited an advanced system of medicine. They described three hundred surgical procedures; created texts on psychiatry, obstetrics, and toxicology; and developed a seven-year training program for healers well before the modern medical school was conceived.

Remarkably, all of this sprang from their fertile minds thousands of years before the invention of the microscope or the adoption of blood work as a trusted diagnostic tool. The ancient rishis, according to historical accounts, cognized the system of Ayurveda through direct contact with nature while in deep meditation. It became an oral tradition passed down from generation to generation. Ayurveda is said to be knowledge based in truth, unchanging, timeless, and eternal—in contrast with modern medicine, which is based on the changing winds of empirical research. (Keep in mind that Ayurveda is not static either; it adapts to new information but hews to its core principles.)

The origins of Ayurveda are shrouded in mystery. No one knows for sure when the first Ayurvedic texts, called the *shastras,* were written, although most experts point to 1000 BCE. These foundational works include a number of books, such as the Charaka Samhita, the Sushruta Samhita, and the Bhagavata Purana. They present Ayurvedic concepts in *sutras,* "threads," of knowledge.

The name *Ayurveda* itself gives us clues about the nature of the system. *Veda* means "science"—science that is built on *siddhantas,* fundamental unchanging principles. *Veda* refers to guided knowledge; it is not just a theory but a road map for how to derive practical benefits from the teachings.

What is *ayu*? Bhava Mishra, a sixteenth-century ancestor of my teacher, Dr. Rama Kant Mishra, compiled a text called the Bhava Prakasha. In it he wrote that ayu means "life"—specifically, what is good and bad for life in terms of diet, nature, behavior, or season.

The Charaka Samhita describes *ayu* in the *sutra deha prana samyoge ayuh,* "*prana* as the life force." In other words, as the reception, flow, and use of prana is reduced in the body, in the cellular system, or in a specific organ or gland, that area becomes compromised, leading to increased inflammation and the gradual failure of the immune system. This is how disease takes root and progresses.

WHAT IS PRANA?

Since good health depends on the balanced flow of prana in the body, it is important to understand its definition. Prana can be found in the food we eat, the air we breathe, the water we drink, and the herbs we take. Prana is that vibration of nature that delivers intelligence to every cell in our bodies. At this deep cellular level, all parts of the body are in communication with each other, and the body at any point in time is performing highly intelligent activities: it is making hormones when it recognizes that they are too low; the cells are making ATP (adenosine triphosphate) for energy; the Krebs cycle is taking place; neurotransmitters are being made. How does the body instinctively know how to do all of this? The initial impulse to perform all these thousands of functions comes from this vibration of nature—provided that we don't destroy it.

If we put chlorine in water, it will kill the prana; the water will be less "intelligent." We can filter the water, but we cannot bring the prana back to life. That is why we do not recommend drinking tap water or filtered water. We also do not recommend drinking water that contains synthetic vitamins or is "electrolyte enhanced" to increase its pH. The water naturally coming from the earth in a pristine environment will automatically have an alkaline pH and nature's life-giving vibration.

Likewise, processing food kills its prana. Processed foods have been stripped of their natural whole nature, leaving them both nutritionally and energetically deficient. Heating food in a microwave superimposes a man-made artificial vibration onto that food, disrupting the prana and rendering it lifeless. Freezing and canning also alter this life force. The ancients went so far as to observe that once cooked, food retained its pranic value for only four hours. Thus, eating leftovers was discouraged.

Ayurvedic herbs are picked and processed according to strict standards laid out in the shastras to keep their prana intact. If their prana is disrupted in any way due to mishandling, the herbs will not work as well, if at all. Taking that concept further, we can see why pharmaceuticals and nutraceuticals, which are made in labs and therefore devoid of the natural vibrational energy of prana, can stress the body, even if they also have positive effects. As these unintelligent chemicals infiltrate the body, they are immediately registered as toxins, causing the liver and kidneys to work overtime as they attempt to process them out of the body.

Notice how happy people are outdoors in nature, whether at the beach, hiking on a mountain path, or simply enjoying a quiet moment at a park. Here, the fresh air they breathe is filled with prana, and they are bolstering their own energy supply with every lungful. Conversely, notice how stressed or drained people look when they are confined in a man-made environment, whether at their desk in an office, walking along a busy city street, or even on the couch in front of the TV. Here, the pranic value of the air is corrupted not just by chemical pollution but also by EMFs (electromagnetic frequencies) from computers, cell phones, Wi-Fi networks, power lines, and so on. EMFs interfere with prana's vibrational signature, creating havoc in the body because it is from this primordial vibration that all the cells of the body emerge. This is why radiation can cause cellular mutations and cancers.

Air, water, and foods that are devoid of prana can be considered "dumb" or "dead," having lost their intelligent vibration. In the long run, if our food, air, and water lack prana, our own cells become dumb in their functions. This is how serious diseases such as autoimmune diseases and cancer take hold. What is cancer? It is cells that have lost their contact with nature—dumb cells that can't remember what they are supposed to be doing and instead create abnormal growths and structures.

One of the basic tenets of this book is that we should all eat good food, drink pure water, get out in nature, and take only those supplements that have good prana to ensure excellent health.

The Three Components of Prana

Prana is composed of three elements: *soma, agni,* and *marut.*

The source of soma is the moon. It is the cooling, nurturing, stabilizing, and growth-giving component of pranic energy.

The source of agni is the sun. It is the fiery component of prana, and as such the source of transformation, responsible for transforming soma, the raw material of nature, into the various parts and systems of the body.

Marut is that energy coming out of the elements of space and air. It is the seed of all five elements (space, air, fire, water, and earth) and contains everything—all of the intelligence of creation. Marut circulates soma inside and outside the body. It is the intelligence-giving component of pranic energy, responsible for organizing the various systems of the body. Marut determines how soma is transformed into the various tissues, neurotransmitters, and hormones and how it interacts with all of these elements.

To give an analogy: when we cook rice, the flame is the agni, the rice and water are the soma, the thermostat is the modulation of the flame, and stirring and mixing of the rice into the water is the marut.

WHAT ARE THE THREE DOSHAS?

All of creation arises from a silent field of pure absolute being. It is unmanifest and unknowable, but it contains the seed within itself, the seed of everything. This seed is called *swara,* which transforms into the primordial sound (*aum*). The primordial sound is the origin from which all of creation manifests. It's a sound vibration that creates matter. This sound vibration is called the *aditattwa.* The aditattwa manifests as the *tritattwa* (or the three primal energies, known as soma, agni, and marut), which then expresses itself as the *panchamahabhutas,* which are space, air, fire, water, and earth, known as the five elements. The vibration of marut becomes the more physical element of space and air, the vibration of agni becomes the more physical element of fire, and the vibration of soma becomes the more physical vibration of water and earth. Notice here that the creation of these elements goes from the most subtle, which is space, to the most solid element of earth. This is how all of creation sequentially unfolds and manifests itself.

To summarize, prana is the cosmic components of tritattwa, flowing together in our bodies and all of creation, manifesting physically as the three doshas—vata, pitta, and kapha—which govern all aspects of our body and mind. Thus, the three doshas are the physical manifestations of the vibrational raw material that is prana and demonstrate how our physical bodies connect to the vibration of cosmic intelligence.

Vata

Vata is the marut-predominant dosha, comprising the elements of space and air and relating to movement, change, and irregularity. It is considered rough, dry, cold, quick, light, and moving. It therefore controls all movement in the body and mind—movement or circulation of the blood, movement of thoughts through the mind, movement of food through the digestive tract, and so on.

Vata types are usually thin, having a hard time keeping weight on due to their all-pervasive restlessness. They are by nature lively, enthusiastic, and creative. Their hair is fine in nature, and they exhibit delicate features in general.

When imbalanced, vata can cause cold hands and feet. Vata types may feel anxious and scattered, endlessly talking and moving, making it difficult to stay focused. Because their nervous system cannot settle down, they may sleep lightly or experience insomnia. Vata is rough and dry, so they may also notice rough and dry hair, skin, and nails. It is very common for a vata type to tap their fingers, pull their hair, and develop all types of tics. Due to too much dryness, their joints tend to crack, and they might even develop a habit of continually popping their joints to relieve the buildup of air in the joint capsules. They may become forgetful as thoughts both come in and leave quickly. Vertigo, restless legs, constipation, and irregular appetite are other common symptoms they may experience throughout their lives.

Pitta

Pitta is the agni-predominant dosha, containing the fire and water elements and relating to metabolism, digestion, and enzymatic processes. It is considered hot, sharp, penetrating, light, liquid, sour, and oily. It is responsible for vision, hunger, the digestion and transformation of food, the regulation of heat in the body, and luster in the complexion.

Pitta types are generally medium in height, and they tend to have moles or freckles, fair skin, blond or red hair, and blue eyes. Their hair may go gray or white prematurely. Thinning of the hair and baldness is also common. Since pitta governs digestion, they usually have a strong metabolism, good digestion, and a healthy appetite. They tend to sweat excessively, and their body temperature may run slightly high, with warm hands and feet. Because of their tendency to overheat, they do not tolerate hot summer days or too much heat in the room.

When imbalanced, pitta can cause ulcers, acid reflux, and excessive heat in the system manifesting as anger, hot flashes, or rashes and various other skin conditions.

Kapha

Kapha, the soma-predominant dosha, contains the earth and water elements and is related to structure and fluid balance. It is cold, damp, dense, heavy, oily, slow, sweet, and stable. Kapha provides stability to both the physical structure and psychological nature.

Kapha types tend to be overweight; their bodies are earthy and heavy with a strong build and stamina. Their hair is usually very thick, dark, and wavy. The whites of their eyes are very white and large. In nature, kapha represents the elements of slowness, so these people are slow and methodical, with slow speech and a calm, thoughtful, and loving mind.

When imbalanced, kapha can cause lethargy, a tendency toward obesity, diabetes, fluid retention, and congestion. Their stable minds, when out of balance, can become resistant to change and tend to cling to the status quo, even if the circumstances are no longer life supporting or necessary.

Balancing the Doshas

We are all born with all three doshas, but in differing ratios. Some people are born with a high amount of vata and less pitta and kapha. We can call them a "vata type." Some might have a greater percentage of vata and pitta and a lot less kapha, and therefore we would consider them a "vata-pitta type." The various combinations could be:

Pure Doshas

Vata

Pitta

Kapha

Dosha Combinations

Vata-pitta	Vata-kapha
Pitta-vata	Pitta-kapha
Kapha-vata	Kapha-pitta

Balance of All Doshas

Vata-pitta-kapha

The balance of the three doshas that you are born with is considered your *prakriti,* your basic nature or constitution. Since it is genetic, your prakriti remain constant for your entire life. However, the manifestation of the doshic energies will change as various influences in the environment and other stressors throw your body out of balance. The imbalances you are currently holding on to, disrupting the three doshas, are considered your *vikruti.*

The word *dosha* means "that which is out of balance" or "that which is in the process of maintaining the body." The doshas are always in action within the body and mind, and by their very nature they disrupt easily. For example, when we get hungry, the pitta dosha goes out of balance—we feel hunger pangs or become lightheaded or weak. The solution to balancing pitta? Eat! As the doshas fall out of balance, we reflexively bring them back into balance by eating, drinking, moving, resting, and all the other normal routines of our day. However, if we fail to recalibrate these three doshas—if we do not maintain proper diet, exercise, and daily routines, along with an uplifted mind and good spiritual path—over time the chronic imbalance can result in disease.

To stay healthy, it is important to keep the doshas in balance. So, for example, if you are a vata type, in order to prevent aggravation of your vata nature, you must learn to slow down; get proper rest; stay warm; eat warm, cooked, unctuous foods; and resist the temptation to go to bed late, work too hard, or exercise too much.

Pitta types, since they have a strong digestive fire, need to eat on time, never skip or delay meals, and avoid hot spicy foods, coffee, and alcohol, which could heat them up more. They have to keep their bodies cool in the summer, protecting their skin and eyes from excessive sunlight.

Kapha types, on the other hand, need to exercise more, eat less, and wake up early and start moving to prevent dullness, lethargy, and laziness from setting in.

THE NINE STAGES OF DISEASE

Disease builds in the body through nine stages. The first two stages show no symptoms. In the third and fourth stages we can have symptoms, but no diagnosable disease. By the fifth and sixth stages, the disease is recognizable. In stages seven through nine, the disease becomes serious and life threatening.

The goal of medicine should be to diagnose and treat disease when it is in the early stages. Nevertheless, modern doctors are trained to use diagnostic tools that detect disease only once it has progressed to a serious level. I see hundreds of patients every year who complain bitterly of their symptoms. They have seen doctors and had diagnostic tests, but they are told that nothing is wrong with them. These patients usually are in the third and fourth stages, where symptoms manifest but a diagnosis cannot be made. This is especially true of thyroid disorders—you can have all the symptoms of thyroid disease, yet your hormone levels fall within normal limits on blood work. Unfortunately, once thyroid disease has progressed to the fifth and sixth stages, where it can be diagnosed by blood work, the patient has already suffered damage. However, even at this stage it may still be possible to repair the thyroid gland without the use of pharmaceutical intervention.

In contrast, the healers of ancient India developed a sophisticated system of pulse diagnosis to detect the earliest inklings of a disease process, which is invaluable for patients and doctors alike, since it is much easier to prevent a disease from developing than to reverse one that is well under way.

Let's take a look at the nine stages, known as the *samprapti chakra,* or "wheel" of pathogenesis, continuing with the example of the imbalanced pitta dosha that in its earliest manifestation shows up simply as hunger. The following explanation derives from the Charaka Samhita.

Stage 1: Accumulation or Sanchaya
In this first stage, if we are hungry and eat, we pacify the accumulation of pitta dosha.

Stage 2: Aggravation or Prakopa
However, if we don't eat, the elevated pitta dosha becomes aggravated. If we eat now, we can still pacify this dosha.

Stage 3: Spread or Prasara
If we fail to eat, skipping and delaying meals on a regular basis, the aggravated pitta dosha starts spreading out to enter the *dhatus* (the tissues) and *malas* (waste products).

Stage 4: Deposition or Localization of Toxins or Sthana Samshraya
If the pitta imbalance continues, toxins are deposited or localized in the dhatus and malas. In these third and fourth stages, the patient will start to manifest symptoms, such as heartburn, a burning sensation during urination, or rectal itching.

Stage 5: Manifestation or Vyakti
In the fifth phase of pathogenesis, the aggravated dosha manifests as blockages in the physical channels and the gaps between the cells and tissues, disturbing the flow, distribution, transformation, and delivery of prana.

Stage 6: Differentiation of Disease or Bheda

Now we see destruction in the body's organs and systems, with structural changes in the physiology. In the case of aggravated pitta, the pitta dosha might invade the wall of the stomach, creating a gastric ulcer that now starts to bleed or perforate.

Stages 7–9: Deformity, Final Disease Symptoms, and Disease Complications or Virupaka, Rogalakshana and Paribhaashaa, and Kledu

From here the imbalanced dosha continues to wreak havoc in the physiology, causing different types of deformity (stage 7), the final symptoms of the disease (stage 8), and complications (stage 9) of that disease. In our example of aggravated pitta, perhaps that perforated or bleeding ulcer now becomes peritonitis, a potentially fatal infection of the abdominal wall, or a gastric cancer that metastasizes to other organs and systems.

THE SEVEN DHATUS (TISSUES)

When we eat food, it travels through the digestive tract and is then absorbed into the bloodstream. From there, it slowly makes its way through the dhatus, or seven tissues:

1. Blood plasma (*rasa*)
2. Blood (*rakta*)
3. Muscle (*mamsa*)
4. Fat (*meda*)
5. Bone (*asthi*)
6. Bone marrow (*majja*)
7. Reproductive fluids (*shukra*)

This sequence is important for many reasons. First, each tissue transforms into the next down the line, which means that the previous tissue needs to be well nourished so that the next tissue is fully developed and strong. So, for example, if you eat a very low-fat diet, then not only will your fat tissue be malnourished but your bone tissue will suffer as well, as the fat tissue provides the raw materials for the formation of bone tissue. This will become an important factor to consider when we discuss two of the symptoms of hypothyroidism: hair loss and osteoporosis. Hair health and growth depend on the nourishment of bone tissue. In fact, hair loss is a symptom of weak bones, and in order for the bone tissue to be nourished you need an ample amount of good-quality fat in your diet (more on that later).

When toxins enter the body, they tend to want to travel the same route, starting at the blood plasma and passing slowly into the next six tissues. When toxins are present in blood plasma and blood, the body tries to excrete them in bowel movements and urine. However, if the body is unable to eliminate them, eventually they travel deep into the bone marrow. Bone marrow is a vital part of the immune system, and toxins here can cause autoimmune tendencies, which will come into play when we discuss Hashimoto's thyroiditis, an autoimmune disease of the thyroid gland.

When all seven tissues are well nourished, the body makes *ojas;* that is, neurotransmitters and hormones. On the other hand, if the tissues are not well nourished, whether from poor diet, weak digestion, or some other condition, then the seven tissues are malnourished and the body produces insufficient ojas—another important factor to consider as we discuss thyroid hormone problems.

Again, this brings us to the inadequacies of Western medicine. When modern diagnostic tests point to low hormone levels, doctors tend to immediately prescribe hormone treatments without consideration of other factors. If the cause of a patient's low hormone levels is weak digestion or deficient diet, then the hormone treatments may correct hormone levels, but the patient will continue to suffer as the root of the imbalance continues to fester. A more comprehensive and holistic diagnosis and treatment is required to bring the patient back to a balanced state of health.

OJAS: NEUROTRANSMITTERS AND HORMONES

Ojas, that vital life force that governs hormonal balance, is considered to be the essence of the seven dhatus. As the final product of our reproductive fluids (shukra), it is also the first element of our body. As the Charaka Samhita notes, "Ojas is the first thing in the body to be developed since it is transmitted to the embryo along with semen and ovum during fertilization. It is like ghee in color, like honey in taste, and like puffed rice in odor."

Ojas gives strength to our physiology and bolsters our immunity to disease. If we have adequate levels of ojas (which can be felt in the pulse), then both chronic and acute disease are less likely. Mother's milk promotes ojas, which is why babies should be breastfed; the milk confers strong immunity to disease. The consumption of ghee (clarified butter) also promotes the formation of ojas. In Western terms, all the steroid hormones of the adrenal glands and the reproductive glands are made from cholesterol. Thus, ghee, which contains good quality cholesterol, provides the essential raw material for the production of these hormones. This information will become important later as we discuss the role of diet in strengthening thyroid (and hormonal) function.

We can also make ojas when we are happy and blissful—when we meditate, pray, chant, or do anything else that gives us joy and happiness. In the same way that our bodies produce serotonin when we are happy, so too do we make ojas.

Optimum levels of ojas give proper nourishment to the body, good body structure and support, great strength, and immunity to disease, as well as optimal hormonal levels and balanced neurotransmitter production. Overexercising, fasting, anxiety, rushing through the day, staying up late, grief, injuries, old age, and excessive discharge of mucus, blood, semen, and other waste products can cause depleted ojas.

THE VIBRATIONAL AND PHYSICAL CHANNELS

The ancient texts described two types of "channels," as they are called. Vibrational channels (*nadis*) carry prana throughout the body, while the physical channels (*srotas*) carry various types of fluids, like urine, sweat, toxins, tears, and so on.

The Vibrational Channels (Nadis)

Prana comes in at the top of the head through the *adhipati marma* point. Marma points are points on the body where prana can be delivered to a specific organ, gland, or cellular system. The adhipati point is found in the area where newborn babies have a fontanel, or soft spot. *Adhipati* means "governing," and this point receives and governs the flow of prana into the body. This is why it is so dangerous to sustain a serious blow to the top of the head—it disrupts this vital flow of life-giving prana to the whole body.

From the adhipati marma point, prana travels down the spine via the *ida* and *pingala* channels. Can you picture the logo of the American Medical Association? It shows these two channels moving up the spine as two snakes intertwined, moving upward around a staff. These vibrational channels receive and deliver prana through the left and right nostrils, with soma-predominant prana coming through the *ida nadi* via the left nostril and agni-predominant prana coming through the *pingala nadi* via the right nostril, mixing in with marut-predominant prana coming down the *shushumna nadi* (spine).

At different times of the day the body requires different ratios of the cooling lunar energy of soma versus the heating solar energy of agni. Thus the right and left flows through the nostrils will shift throughout the day, allowing more soma in the early morning hours to build stamina and strength (soma is the raw material to make kapha and ojas), preparing the body for its busy day, for example, or allowing more agni after eating, when the body needs more agni to digest food.

Yogic breathing techniques, known as *pranayama,* balance the reception and delivery of all three pranic energies—soma, agni, and marut—as well as the ida, pingala, and shushumna nadis, delivering these energies wherever they are needed within the body.

There are other nadis that receive prana as well, such as the *gandhari* (left eye), *hastijihva* (right eye), *yasavini* (left ear), *alambusa* (right ear), and *loma rondhra* (hair follicles of the skin over the entire body). The flow of prana from all of these orifices circulates down the spine and is delivered to all the organs and systems, eventually flowing out through the hands and feet.

When pranic flow is normal, the doshas that govern our body and mind are balanced. When pranic flow is obstructed, however, disease begins. Pranic obstructions can result from EMFs, injuries, surgical scars, and misalignments of the spine, among other things

The Physical Channels (Srotas)

Once food is broken down in the gastrointestinal tract and absorbed into the bloodstream, it flows through the various physical channels until it comes out the other end as a bowel movement, urine, sweat, tears, and so on.

If these physical channels become shrunken, inflamed, clogged, or hardened, the passage of fluids is disrupted, creating problems for the body. Nicotine from cigarettes, for example, can shrink the arteries, one of the physical channels, which can contribute to heart disease because less blood is able to reach the heart muscle. Ulcerative colitis is an example of a physical channel (the intestines) becoming inflamed, with ulcers forming as the immune system mounts its attack on the delicate intestinal lining.

Have you ever noticed that breastfed babies have fewer ear infections than formula-fed babies? This is because breast milk is very light and absorbs easily into cells, whereas the formulas are dense and thick, clogging the baby's delicate channels. If the food coming in clogs the initial channel (the gastrointestinal tract), all subsequent channels (including the ear canals) will clog. As the food sits stuck and semidigested in the ear channels, it begins to breed infection.

You can actually rupture the physical channels with improper and overzealous cleansing techniques. If you attempt to pull out highly acidic toxins (such as years of birth control pills) too quickly, the acids can rupture the channels as they exit through the bowel, urinary, and sweat channels. This is why I recommend preparing and lubricating the physical channels before a detox program, and once detoxification is initiated, it is important to bind the toxins and direct them carefully and slowly out of the body. Thus it is very important that you undertake detoxification with a practitioner who is familiar with the correct way to remove toxins, and let him or her monitor you through the whole detox process.

Chapter 8 describes the best diet and daily routine to prevent clogging, shrinking, inflaming, or hardening of the physical channels, and we'll talk more about cleansing techniques in chapter 3.

PULSE DIAGNOSIS

The ancient healers of Ayurveda developed a system of pulse diagnosis, called *nadi vigyan*. The pulse is felt in the artery, a physical channel or srota, but within that artery is the nadi, the vibrational channel. Thus, though pulse assessment focuses on the physical artery, it is primarily an examination of pranic flow. Since prana orchestrates the smooth functioning of our body at all levels—every cell, organ, and gland needs a constant supply of prana—it is important to know whether the flow of prana is normal or obstructed, the latter a sign of developing or advanced disease.

The pulse diagnosis taught in Ayurveda bears no resemblance to the pulse diagnosis used in modern medicine. Western practitioners learn to read the rate and rhythm of the pulse—how many times per minute your heart is beating and whether there is regular rhythm. Ayurvedic practitioners, in contrast, use the pulse to access very deep information about how the whole physiology is functioning, from the organs, glands, and seven tissues to the doshas, vibrational channels, and physical channels. One can also feel the four different types of toxins (see chapter 3) and which tissues they have deposited in. Pulse diagnosis enables Ayurvedic practitioners to detect the very early stages of the disease process, sometimes years before it becomes apparent.

Feeling the Seven Tissues in the Pulse

In the first level of the pulse you can detect information on the first tissue, rasa (blood plasma). Did the patient digest her food properly, or is it stuck in the channel, clogging it, due to heavy food or poor digestion?

In the second level you can feel the vibration of rakta (blood tissue).

What types of toxins are sitting in there? How is the flow? Is the blood hot or cool?

In the third level you can feel any imbalances in the mamsa (muscle tissue). Are toxins present, which could cause fibromyalgia? Did the patient take a statin drug that has gone to the muscle tissue, weakening and disturbing its normal function?

In the fourth level of the pulse you can detect the quality of meda (fat tissue). Is the patient eating poor-quality vegetable oil, such as canola, and depositing free radicals into the fat tissue? Is the patient consuming a low-fat diet and starving this tissue of proper nourishment?

In the fifth level you can detect the health and strength of asthi (bone tissue). Has the patient been avoiding healthy fats, thus depleting this tissue and potentially causing osteopenia or osteoporosis?

At the sixth level you can feel the integrity of majja (bone marrow). Has the patient stored toxins from air pollution, pesticides, heavy metals, or pharmaceuticals, which are now stuck in his bone marrow and upsetting immune function? This situation can lead to autoimmune tendency or cancer.

The seventh level reveals the strength of shukra (reproductive fluids). Are these tissues weak and malnourished because any one of the tissues preceding them were also weak?

Feeling the Strength, Rhythm, and Volume in the Pulse

In the middle range of pulse diagnosis, somewhere between the first and the seventh tissues, you can determine the overall strength (*bala*), rhythm (*laya*), and volume (*poornata*) of the pulse.

Bala: Strength

Bala is not just physical strength; it also refers to the mental, emotional, physical, and sensual strengths of the individual. There are three levels of bala: optimal (*balvati*), medium (*nirbala*), and weak (*durbala*).

Laya: Rhythm

Laya, the rhythm of the pulse, is broken down into eight divisions:

1. Balanced and blissful (*sama*)
2. Normal (*sarala*)
3. Exhibiting happiness or "happy bouncing" (*prasanna*)
4. A little out of sync (*niyamita*)
5. Somewhat off, with a few waves out of balance, indicating the beginning of an unhealthy state (*vishama*)
6. Moving in and out in different directions (*vishama gamini*)
7. Completely missing some beats, validating that the body and mind are not connected (*trutika*)
8. Moving in first one direction and then another, showing a complete lack of connection between mind and body (*gati kautilya*); this is an unhealthy rhythm and a very ominous sign

It is common for a weak thyroid to affect the normal rhythm of the pulse, and it is so gratifying to see the rhythm return to normal as the thyroid gland strengthens.

Poornata: Volume

The volume, poornata, of the pulse is categorized in six stages:

1. More than full or overflowing (*sthula*)
2. Perfect volume (*poorna*)
3. Not low; less than optimal (*apoorna*)
4. Significantly less than normal volume (*rikta*)
5. A thready, thin, and weak pulse (*sukshma*); this is an ominous sign
6. A thin, thready, extremely weak pulse (*krishna*) that occurs when a patient is losing a lot of prana or blood or is about to die; it signifies chronic illness with no bala and is a grave sign

The volume of the pulse can be lowered by, among other things, dehydration and poor diet.

Feeling Vata, Pitta, and Kapha in the Pulse

The middle range of the pulse also reveals the strength and integrity of the vata, pitta, and kapha doshas. Is there too much vata, so that the patient is nervous, weak, or spacey? Is pitta aggravated, causing anger, ravenous appetite, or acid reflux? Is kapha imbalanced, creating dullness, lethargy, and depression?

Pulse diagnosis allows us to go even deeper to evaluate the subdoshas; that is, the five specific areas where each primary dosha exerts its unique influence.

THE SUBDOSHAS

The Vata Subdoshas

Prana Vata

Prana vata is located in the region of the head. It governs not only the movement of thoughts through the mind but the flow of intelligence for the entire body. It also governs the other four vata subdoshas, and therefore any treatment geared toward prana vata will automatically balance the other vata subdoshas. If imbalanced, prana vata can cause anxiety and insomnia as your mind incessantly races.

Udana Vata

Udana vata is located in the chest and upward to the throat. It flows upward and governs all of the *karmendriyas,* or the physical organs of action that facilitate our direct contact with the outer world, including those of excretion (anus), procreation (reproductive organs), locomotion (legs), grasping (hands), breathing (lungs), and speech (mouth).

Imbalanced udana vata can manifest in lack of courage (from lack of coordination between the mind, body, and senses). It can also affect your facial complexion, creating a cyanotic color of blue, since insufficient prana in the lungs can result in shallow or difficult breathing and inadequate oxygenation of the blood.

It is also responsible for speech, expression, and enthusiasm. When out of balance, it can lead to speech problems, coughs, sore throat, and throat infections.

Quite often it is this subdosha that vibrates out of balance if there is a problem with the thyroid, as the thyroid gland is located in the region governed by udana vata (the throat).

Samana Vata

Samana vata is located in the stomach and governs the clockwise churning of food as it is processed in the stomach. *Samana* means "balancing," and this subdosha balances the other vata subdoshas: prana, udana, *vyana,* and *apana.* It also balances the peristalsis of the small and large intestine, helping the processes of digestion, assimilation, and absorption. If it falls out of balance, it can cause gas in the stomach and upward pressure, leading to belching and hiccups.

Vyana Vata

Vyana vata is located in the heart and governs the circulation of blood. It governs the reflex actions of the autonomic nervous system—for example, blinking your eyes when you are startled. An imbalance here can lead to problems associated with poor circulation and high blood pressure.

Apana Vata

Apana vata, located in the pelvic region, controls impulses related to urination, elimination, and menstruation. Apana is a downward flow of energy, responsible for bringing the menstrual fluid down, the bowel movement and urine down and out, and even babies downward during delivery. Apana is also responsible for releasing the body's used-up prana through all the channels of elimination.

If your mind is overactive, apana can mistakenly flow upward, disturbing the digestive organs on its way up and thus causing problems with digestion (like acid reflux, gas, gastroparesis, hiatal hernias, and bloating), hiccups, endometriosis (as the blood flows upward and spills into the pelvic cavity), menstrual cramps, constipation, long labor, and low back pain. Apana can also fall out of balance if you are overactive (excessive movement and stress on the pelvis and legs) or sedentary (insufficient movement of the pelvis and legs). Even wearing constrictive clothing around the waist can cause imbalance of this subdosha.

Disturbance of apana vata is rampant in our fast-paced society, and it is responsible for numerous hormonal imbalances in women, since it is located in the region of the ovaries.

The Pitta Subdoshas

Pachaka Pitta

Pachaka pitta is located in the stomach and small intestine and facilitates the digestion of food. It is described as the flame that burns up food; if this flame is too high, it can create gastritis or ulcers.

Ranjaka Pitta

Ranjaka pitta resides in the liver and spleen. *Ranjaka* derives from *ranjan*, "coloring," and refers to that which gives color to our blood plasma, or *rasa dhatu*. Rasa is formed after the initial stage of digestion. Then ranjaka pitta transforms the plasma to make blood. Ranjaka pitta is the fuel for the liver and has five flames, or *agnis*, in order to process and transform the five elements that come from food: space, air, fire, water, and earth.

This subdosha is commonly out of balance today because the liver gets overloaded attempting to handle toxins from processed foods, pharmaceuticals, nutraceuticals, pesticides, air pollution, and toxins from various skin-care products that leach through the skin and immediately wind up in the blood.

Sadhaka Pitta

Sadhaka pitta is found in the heart and brain. It is the emotional pitta that helps us transform or digest our emotional challenges. Inflammation is created throughout the body as our negative thoughts and feelings imbalance this subdosha. If left untreated, it can develop into depression.

Alochaka Pitta

Alochaka pitta is located in the eyes and helps us see and feel, affecting not just physical sight but also perception from the depths of our consciousness, which is why we close our eyes when meditating or in prayer. Imbalances in this subdosha are connected to eye problems.

Bhrajaka Pitta

Bhrajaka pitta is located in the skin. This subdosha governs our complexion, particularly the skin's color and aura. When it is out of balance, we can suffer from skin conditions such as eczema, psoriasis, and itching or burning rashes.

The Kapha Subdoshas

Tarpaka Kapha

Tarpaka kapha is found in the lubricant/fluid surrounding the brain and spinal cord. When the brain becomes dried out by excessive prana vata (aggravation from too much stress), tarpaka kapha is the protective mechanism that comes to lubricate and nourish the brain. Tarpaka functions to support memory and prevent dementia. It also governs the myelin sheath, which coats and insulates our nerves and is essential for proper functioning of our nervous system. As discussed previously, marut-predominant prana runs from the adhipati marma point on the top of the head and then down the spinal column. Marut is composed of space and air, so it has a tendency to be drying. Thus the spinal cord needs constant lubrication, cooling, and nourishment. Disturbance in tarpaka kapha can lead to multiple sclerosis and other demyelinating diseases.

Bodhaka Kapha

Bodhaka kapha governs our taste buds and allows us to perceive the six tastes (sweet, sour, salty, pungent, bitter, and astringent). When it is out of balance, we are unable to perceive taste correctly. It also protects the oral cavity by supplying saliva when it is dry. Dry mouth, receding gums, and gum infections are all signs of low bodhaka kapha.

Kledaka Kapha

Kledaka kapha is located within the mucosal lining of the gastro-intestinal tract. It lubricates the food we put into our mouths and keeps it moist in our stomachs so it can churn properly and prevent pachaka pitta from burning the mucous membranes. When kledaka kapha is low, gas, distension, burning pain in the stomach, and ulcers can occur.

Avalambaka Kapha

Avalambaka kapha, is located in the chest. *Avalambaka* means "depending on," or "to hold or support," referring to the fact that we are mentally, physically, and emotionally dependent on it for a solid foundation. When this subdosha is out of balance, we lose our mental stability, creating a feeling of hopelessness, a decline in faith, and a persistently negative attitude.

Shleshaka Kapha

Shleshaka kapha is present in the synovial fluid of the joints. It nourishes and lubricates the articular surfaces and promotes flexibility of the joints. It also lubricates the capillaries and skin, as well as the gaps between organs, the gaps between cells, and even the gaps between DNA and RNA molecules—any physical gap where two things are connected and working together. Abnormalities of this subdosha can lead to osteoarthritis and other structural damage to the joints.

As you can see, the pulse is a valuable detailed blueprint of a patient's health, giving practitioners quick access to both current and past information regarding the patient's body, mind, soul, and spirit. It can detect the very early stages of the disease process, when intervention is critical to prevent full-blown disease, and it can also serve as an excellent tool for monitoring patient progress during treatment.

Despite all the Sanskrit terms and complicated bodily interactions

I have described in this chapter, regaining or maintaining your health boils down to common sense, which is the essence of Ayurveda. Thus your prescription for attaining perfect health is straightforward and simple: eat when you are hungry, drink when you are thirsty, sleep when you are tired. Simple as that.

2

The Thyroid Gland
and Endocrine System

" " Judy, please follow me back to the treatment room." Walking with my next patient, I noticed her wiping tears from her eyes. As we sat down to discuss her case history, I grabbed some tissues for her to use as she told her story. She detailed her symptoms: hair falling out in chunks to the point where she had to wear a wig; weight gain no matter how little she ate or how many hours she spent each week in the gym, working out next to skinny women—which sent her self-esteem plummeting; heart skipping beats as she lay in bed at night wondering whether she might suffer a heart attack; and brain fog. As I took her case history I found myself finishing sentences for her as she struggled to remember even the most mundane words. Her legs and ankles were swollen, and she felt depressed each day even though she has a terrific husband and wonderful children.

To make matters worse, she told me, all of her lab tests were normal. Her thyroid was normal, and her colonoscopy and blood work were fine. The only problems her doctors had identified were that her cholesterol was a little high and her vitamin D was a little low. So she was left with no options other than to exercise more, eat less, and take antidepressants to elevate her mood. She tried them and gained forty pounds.

Judy is not alone. Hers is a typical case that I see several times a day all week long, year after year. Western medicine seems to be generally unhelpful for these patients. When blood work analyses of thyroid function show normal function, these patients, who are experiencing thyroid deficiency but have not yet progressed to the level of diagnosable disease, are left to suffer. And when thyroid hormones test too low, doctors usually simply prescribe the synthetic thyroid hormone levothyroxine (Levothroid, Synthroid, Levoxyl). As an alternative, some doctors recommend the more natural forms of thyroid hormone made from desiccated pig thyroid glands (such as Armour Thyroid, Nature-Throid, and Westhroid). Yet when I see patients taking either of these two types of thyroid medications, not much has changed, and their symptoms continue.

Some holistic doctors recommend nutraceuticals to support the thyroid gland. However, nutraceuticals are synthetic versions of the nutrients found in food, herbs, and spices, and while they may have a benefit and alleviate some symptoms, they also come with a number of side effects and are harmful to the liver and kidneys in much the same way as pharmaceuticals.

Some Ayurvedic doctors prescribe herbs like ashwagandha, shilajit, and shatavari, which have great benefit for the thyroid and are not toxic to the kidneys or liver. This is a good start, but without taking into account why the thyroid gland is weak in the first place, this treatment too falls short.

Thyroid weakness, or hypothyroidism, usually develops over time due to late bedtime, toxins, intestinal infections, improper diet, overwork or stress, or a genetic predisposition. Using pulse diagnosis (described in chapter 1), not only can we identify weakness in the thyroid gland at a much earlier stage than blood work would reveal, but just as important, we can identify the specific factors that are weakening this very delicate gland in any particular patient.

As early as 1976, Broda O. Barnes, M.D., sounded a warning to the medical community in his groundbreaking book on the subject, *Hypothyroidism: The Unsuspected Illness.* He alerted doctors that thousands of people across the country were suffering weakness in the thyroid but remained undiagnosed and therefore untreated due to the lack of sensitivity of the available thyroid tests.

Since then, numerous books and research articles have been written on the subject of "subclinical" thyroid conditions that do not show up on blood work. Even when doctors suspect a subclinical thyroid condition and prescribe hormones, whether natural or synthetic, nothing much changes for the patient. Why? The thyroid gland only knows to make hormones when it gets a signal from the pituitary gland that thyroid hormone levels are too low. If the patient is taking thyroid hormones, the thyroid gland, which was already malfunctioning, simply goes to sleep. With the body receiving thyroid hormones from an external source, the thyroid gland has no need to produce any. This is why many patients need more and more supplementary thyroid hormone as the years go by.

Remember Judy? She had been prescribed natural thyroid hormones, iodine, tyrosine, and ashwagandha, yet she had experienced no relief. This is because her treatment was geared mainly toward correcting thyroid hormone insufficiencies, when there are many other factors to consider.

To understand what those other factors are and how we can effectively address hypothyroidism at the level of its root cause, we must first understand the function of the thyroid gland and its role in physiology, including its relationship with the rest of the endocrine system. Let's take a look.

THE ENDOCRINE SYSTEM

The thyroid is part of the endocrine system, which is composed of glands and organs that produce, store, and release hormones into the bloodstream. The hormones travel in the bloodstream throughout the body until they meet up with their target site.

Hormones regulate the function of every cell of the body. But to activate a response, a hormone has to attach to a specific receptor site on a cell's membrane. The membrane is a thin barrier that surrounds and encloses the cell. It is semipermeable, which means that it allows certain substances into the cell while keeping other substances out. Different cells have receptor sites for different hormones, and those receptor sites function in what is often described as a lock-and-key mechanism. If the key (a hormone) fits the lock (the receptor site), then the door in the cell membrane opens and an effect takes place.

Each gland in the endocrine system is responsible for secreting specific kinds of hormones, which in turn stimulate specific responses in the physiology.

Pineal Gland

The pineal gland is located near the center of the brain. Unlike the rest of the brain, it is not isolated from the rest of the body by the blood-brain barrier. Though its function was unknown until recent times, mystical and esoteric traditions referred to this area in the middle of the brain as the connecting link between the physical and spiritual realms.

The pineal gland is the source of melatonin, a hormone derived from tryptophan. It regulates our circadian rhythms by producing more melatonin in the absence of light and decreasing its production in the presence of light. Special photoreceptor cells in the retina detect the presence or absence of light and send signals via the hypothalamus to the pineal gland to regulate melatonin production. Melatonin production therefore peaks during the nighttime hours, enabling us to sleep by slowing down our bodily processes, and is lowest during the daytime, helping us feel alert and ready to take on the day's challenges.

So to get the most benefits from sleep and your melatonin cycle, make sure your room is totally dark at night—don't keep a night-light on, and oh yes, no smart phones next to your head!

One other important point: The timing, length, and frequency of menstrual cycles are influenced by melatonin, so it is important to follow the advice of the ancient seers of India to be asleep when the sun goes down and awake when the sun comes up. In the revolutionary and remarkable book, *The Secret Life of Plants,* researchers demonstrated how animals stop ovulating and become infertile when lights are shined on them at night to keep them awake, effectively illustrating the powerful effects of daylight and darkness on our delicately balanced endocrine systems.

Hypothalamus

The hypothalamus sends hormones to the pituitary gland to signal it to either release or inhibit hormones to the other endocrine glands. When thyroid hormones become too low, for example, the hypothalamus will release thyrotropin-releasing hormone (TRH) to stimulate the pituitary gland to release thyroid-stimulating hormone (TSH), which signals the thyroid gland to ramp up its production of thyroid hormones. It does the same with the gonads, releasing gonadotropin-releasing hormone (GnRH) and, with the adrenals, releasing corticotropin-releasing hormone (CRH).

It also secretes growth hormone–releasing hormone, growth hormone–inhibiting hormone, oxytocin, and antidiuretic hormone. These hormones are then transported to and stored in the posterior part of the pituitary gland until needed. Oxytocin triggers uterine contractions during childbirth and the release of milk during breast-feeding. Antidiuretic hormone prevents water loss in the body by increasing the uptake of water in the kidneys and reducing blood flow to the sweat glands.

Pituitary Gland

The pea-sized pituitary gland is small and oval shaped and is located near the underside of the brain right behind the bridge of the nose. It sits in a small depression in the sphenoid bone, famously called the *sella turcica,* or Turkish saddle, as it closely resembles the saddle of a horse. It is made of two separate structures, the posterior and anterior pituitary glands.

The posterior pituitary is actually composed of nerve tissue, not glandular tissue, and stores and releases oxytocin and antidiuretic hormone as needed.

The anterior pituitary is the true glandular part of the pituitary gland. Its function is under the control of the various releasing and inhibiting hormones sent to it by the hypothalamus. It manufactures six hormones:

- Thyroid-stimulating hormone (TSH), which tells the thyroid gland to produce its hormones
- Adrenocorticotropic hormone (ACTH), which stimulates the adrenal cortex to produce its hormones
- Follicle-stimulating hormone (FSH), which stimulates the gonads to produce eggs in females and sperm in males
- Luteinizing hormone (LH), which stimulates the gonads to produce estrogens in females and testosterone in males
- Human growth hormone (HGH), which affects the growth, repair, and reproduction of many of the cells throughout the body
- Prolactin (PRL), which stimulates the mammary glands of the breasts to produce milk

The pituitary gets information about the levels of hormones circulating in the blood in two ways: by directly detecting the hormone levels on its own and by signals from the hypothalamus.

Thyroid Gland

The thyroid gland affects virtually every cell, organ, and gland in our bodies and, in reverse, can be affected by numerous negative factors in our environment and physiology. The thyroid produces calcitonin, which decreases blood calcium levels when they rise above a certain point. It also produces triiodothyronine (T3) and thyroxine (T4), which together regulate the body's metabolic rate, growth, temperature, heartbeat rate and rhythm, digestive functions, reproductive system, muscle control, brain development, and bone maintenance.

Parathyroid Glands

These four small masses of glandular tissue are found on the posterior side of the thyroid gland and produce parathyroid hormone (PTH) when calcium levels fall too low in the blood. PTH stimulates the osteoclasts (bone cells) to break down calcium and release it into the bloodstream, while at the same time it triggers the kidneys to conserve the calcium that was filtered out of the bloodstream and return it back to the blood rather than releasing it into the urine.

Adrenal Glands

The adrenal glands sit on top of the kidneys and are composed of the outer adrenal cortex and the inner adrenal medulla. The adrenal cortex produces two main groups of corticosteroid hormones: glucocorticoids and mineralocorticoids, as well as androgens.

The glucocorticoids are predominantly cortisol, which helps control the body's use of fats, proteins, and carbohydrates, suppresses inflammation, regulates blood pressure, increases blood sugar, and can also decrease bone formation. It is released during times of stress to help your body get an energy boost and better handle an emergency situation.

The most important mineralocorticoid is aldosterone, which helps control blood pressure by signaling the kidneys to allow sodium to reabsorb into the bloodstream and to release potassium into the urine, thus regulating electrolytes and blood pH.

The androgens that the adrenal cortex produces are dehydroepiandrosterone (DHEA) and testosterone. These hormones are precursor hormones that are converted in the ovaries into female hormones (estrogens) and in the testes into male hormones (androgens).

The adrenal medulla is located inside the adrenal cortex and produces epinephrine and norepinephrine under stimulation by the sympathetic division of the autonomic nervous system. These hormones activate the "fight-or-flight" response to stress. They increase blood flow to the brain and muscles, heart rate, breathing rate, and blood pressure and decrease the flow of blood to and function of organs not involved in that response (like the digestive organs).

Most of women's estrogen (and progesterone) after menopause is produced by the adrenal glands, which is yet another reason to keep your glandular system strong as you age!

Pancreas

The pancreas is a large gland. It is considered a "heterocrine" gland because it contains both endocrine and exocrine tissue. The exocrine part of the pancreas excretes enzymes to break down proteins, fats, carbohydrates, and nucleic acids in food.

The endocrine part of the pancreas accounts for only about 1 percent of the total mass of the organ and is found in small clusters called the islets of Langerhans. These islets contain alpha cells that produce glucagon, which raises blood glucose levels by triggering muscle and liver cells to break down glycogen for the release of glucose into the bloodstream. It also contains beta cells that produce insulin, which lowers blood glucose levels after a meal. Insulin triggers the absorption of glucose from the blood into the cells, where it is added to glycogen molecules for storage. Thus the pancreas controls blood sugar levels throughout the day, increasing and decreasing them as needed.

Gonads

The gonads are the glands that produce sex hormones; that is, the ovaries in females and testes in males.

The testes produce the androgen testosterone after the start of puberty, which causes growth and strengthens bones and muscles. It also contributes to the development of the sex organs and body hair, including pubic, chest, and facial hair.

The ovaries produce progesterone and estrogens. Progesterone is most active in females during ovulation and pregnancy, when it prevents miscarriage. Estrogen promotes the development of the uterus and breasts, pubic and armpit hair, the growth of the bones during adolescence, and the regulation of the menstrual cycle and reproductive system.

Thymus

Found behind the sternum, the thymus gland produces hormones called thymosins that help train and develop T lymphocytes (T cells) during fetal development and childhood, protecting the body from pathogens.

The Skin

The skin, you may ask? Well, technically the skin isn't an endocrine gland but an organ—it's the largest organ in the body, actually. However, the skin also manufactures a hormone: vitamin D. Yes, vitamin D is, in fact, a hormone, not a vitamin. Our skin makes most of the vitamin D that the body requires; only about 10 percent of our vitamin D comes from the food we eat.

Vitamin D is produced in the skin as it absorbs ultraviolet B (UVB) rays. The liver and kidneys are then involved in converting this inactive form of vitamin D into an active form the body can use.

Vitamin D plays a major role in maintaining normal blood levels of calcium and phosphorus. It helps us absorb calcium from the intestines so we can build strong bones. However, as new research has revealed, vitamin D affects more than just bone health. For one thing, vitamin D deficiency can cause low estrogen in women and low testosterone in men, affecting libido. This may be why our libido seems to increase in the spring, stays strong through the summer, and declines somewhat as we go through the winter months.

Other studies have shown that vitamin D activates the genes that release dopamine and serotonin, neurotransmitters that keep us happy and calm. It has also been shown to affect our immune system, which is one reason our immunity declines in the winter months in concert with less sun exposure. A deficiency of vitamin D can also lead to auto-immune diseases, such as multiple sclerosis. Further, decreased levels of vitamin D have been implicated in cancer, heart disease, stroke, and diabetes. Taken altogether, it seems that our understanding of the impact of vitamin D on our physiology is growing every day.

The Kidneys

The kidneys are not usually considered part of the endocrine system, but they do produce the hormone renin, which helps control blood pressure, and the hormone erythropoietin, which stimulates the bone marrow to produce red blood cells.

❧

The endocrine system is like a finely tuned orchestra—problems or weakness in one part of the system can adversely affect other parts of the system. There are many stressors on the endocrine system that we cannot control—workplace stress, accidents and injuries, and so on. But it turns out that we can control these two huge stressors: what time we go to bed and what we eat. If we are disciplined with both, we give our body more leeway to handle the other stressors, making it more difficult for them to drag us down into ill health. We'll talk about both factors in the next chapter.

NOW BACK TO THE THYROID GLAND

The thyroid gland is situated in the throat, just below the Adam's apple. As we noted above, it affects just about every other organ in the body, and it is involved in regulating metabolism, heartbeat rhythm, digestive function, muscle control, brain development, and bone maintenance. It provides hormones for energy production and profoundly affects our moods and emotions.

Here is an amazing fact: Every cell in the body has receptor sites for specific hormones, but only two types of receptor sites are found on *all* cells. What are they? Thyroid hormone and vitamin D receptor sites. What does that indicate? That literally every cell in the body is dependent on a normally functioning thyroid gland! It also accounts for why the thyroid gland responds to every insult in the body. (As for the vitamin D receptors, I suspect that the ubiquity of the receptor sites shows that we are only skimming the surface of what we know about vitamin D's effects on the body; I eagerly await new research revealing more details about this hormone's influence within our bodies.)

When thyroid hormone levels fall too low, the hypothalamus secretes thyrotropin-releasing hormone (TRH), which stimulates the pituitary gland to release thyroid-stimulating hormone (TSH), which signals the thyroid gland to make more hormones. When thyroid hormone levels become too high, TSH levels decrease to signal the thyroid to reduce its production of hormones.

Thyroid hormones are made by attaching iodine molecules to tyrosine, an amino acid. Tyrosine is synthesized in the body from phenylalanine, an amino acid found in many high-protein foods such as chicken, turkey, fish, milk, yogurt, cottage cheese, almonds, sesame seeds, and avocados. (Vegetarians take note: most of the food sources of tyrosine are animal proteins.) Thyroid cells are the only cells in the body that can absorb iodine, which is found in fish, sea vegetables, and various other foods (see chapter 3 for a more comprehensive list).

TSH stimulates thyroid peroxidase (TPO) activity to use iodine to create thyroxine (T4), triiodothyronine (T3), diiodothyronine (T2), and monoiodothyronine (T1) hormones. The numbers 1 through 4 designate the number of iodine molecules attached to the tyrosine molecule: T4 has four iodine molecules, T3 has three molecules, and so on. As a whole, thyroid hormones are 80 percent T4 and 15 percent T3, with the remaining 5 percent divided between T2 and T1.

T4 cannot enter your cells, however. T3, considered the active form of the hormone, is the one that affects metabolism since it can gain entrance into your cells. Not much yet is known about the function of T2 and T1, but I hope future research will give us further clues as to their effects on the body.

Many of my patients ask me why our bodies make so much T4 when it can't be used by our cells. Wouldn't it be more efficient for the thyroid to produce just T3, since it is T3 that does all the work? Good question!

It turns out that yes, the body is wiser than we think. It has a plan and a reason for everything. T4 circulates around the body in the bloodstream and is stored in the tissues, where it lies in wait for that moment when signals are released that more T3 is needed, at which point it comes out of storage and is converted into T3.

Problems with T4 to T3 Conversion
When the body requires T4 to be converted to T3, about 80 percent of the T4 is converted to T3 by the liver, and about 20 percent of the T4

goes to the gastrointestinal tract, where friendly bacteria convert it to T3.

Now consider this: Most of us lack adequate levels of intestinal flora, which are so vital to our digestion, metabolism, and immune system functions. Who among us has never depleted their friendly gut bacteria by taking antibiotics, birth control pills, steroids, or various other pharmaceuticals? You're probably thinking that, yes, while you may have taken these medications, you were diligent enough to take a probiotic afterward or to replenish your gut with your favorite organic yogurt with live probiotic cultures, so you should be okay. However, what you probably don't know is that most of the probiotic cultures on the market are ineffective because most of their cultures die during processing. The same is true of yogurts—they tend to lose their bacterial cultures as they sit on the shelves in the supermarket.

If you haven't been diagnosed with a liver problem, like hepatitis or fatty liver, you may also believe that your liver function is fine and fully capable of converting T4 into T3. You're likely wrong. The liver is ailing in most people. Almost 99 percent of the new patients I see have to do some repair work on their liver. Think of this: everything you have ever swallowed, every chemical you have ever breathed in, and every product you have ever applied to your skin has been processed by your liver. Over time, the liver carries quite a toxic load.

And on top of that, we live in a country that does not recognize the importance of internal cleansing. As a result, the liver is left holding on to many acid toxins, overheats, and cannot perform any of its functions well, including converting T4 into T3. This is a tremendous problem that I see in all of my patients, yet most people—including most doctors—are unaware of it.

Without effectively treating the liver and gut flora, it is nearly impossible to treat any weakness of the thyroid gland, whether it is hypothyroidism or Hashimoto's thyroiditis. For this reason, later in this book we will discuss the herbs used to treat inflammation in the liver and the best sources of prebiotics and probiotics to ensure proper cooling and quick and effective replacement of the friendly bacteria.

Very exciting research focused on this extremely important

conversion of T4 to T3 was published in 2015 by Brock McGregor in which he discusses the fact that it is the peripheral metabolism (metabolism occurring outside of the thyroid gland) which converts T4 to T3 through a number of pathways. His article establishes the numerous factors that can interfere with this conversion, causing patients to experience hypothyroid symptoms even when their thyroid blood tests are normal. These factors include problems with liver and kidney function, inflammation, illness, lifestyle behaviors—including fasting, alcohol dependence and smoking, and depletion of nutrients such as zinc and selenium, to name a few. We will discuss all of these factors and more in upcoming chapters.

Bound versus Free Thyroid Hormones

The thyroid hormones are transported through the bloodstream by thyroid-binding proteins, measured in blood work as thyroid-binding globulins (TBG). These special proteins personally chauffeur the thyroid hormones around the body, dropping them off where needed. Once they are dropped off, they become "free" hormones, labeled in blood work as "free T4" or "free T3." Only the free hormones can exert an influence on the cells of the body, but the body is covetous of its thyroid hormones: about 99 percent of the thyroid hormones are bound. They are freed only as needed. Too much TBG or bound hormones causes active thyroid hormone levels to become low, creating hypothyroidism or underactive thyroid function. Too much free T4 or T3 creates hyperthyroidism or overactive thyroid function. Illnesses, liver diseases, birth control pills, hormone replacement therapy, and corticosteroids (such as prednisone) can affect your TBG levels.

Research published in 2014 by endocrinologist Kent Holtorf in the *Journal of Restorative Medicine* demonstrates "that reduced transport of T4 and T3 into the cells is seen in a variety of common conditions, including insulin resistance, diabetes, depression, bipolar disorder, hyperlipidemia, chronic fatigue syndrome, fibromyalgia, neurodegenerative diseases, migraines, stress, anxiety, chronic dieting, and aging, *while the T3 level in the pituitary often remains unaffected.* The pituitary has different transporters from every other tissue in the body. The thyroid transporters in the body are very energy dependent and are affected by numerous conditions, including low energy states, toxins, and mitochondria dysfunction, while the pituitary remains unaffected" [emphasis added by author].

He goes on to state that "because the pituitary remains largely unaffected and is able to maintain its intracellular (the level of hormone *inside* the cell) T3 levels while the rest of the body suffers from significantly reduced intracellular T3 levels, there is no elevation in thyroid-stimulating hormone (TSH) despite the presence of widespread tissue hypothyroidism, *making the TSH and other standard blood tests a poor marker to determine the presence or absence of hypothyroidism*" [emphasis added by author]. He concludes by emphatically making the case that patients may present with signs and symptoms of hypothyroidism and yet exhibit a normal TSH level, thus warning clinicians to combine both clinical and laboratory assessments to include other parameters, such as Reverse T3 (see below) to make a better determination of thyroid malfunction.

Reverse T3 Formation

Reverse T3 (RT3) is a biologically inactive form of T3. RT3 is a "mirror molecule" of normal T3; it adheres to the same receptor sites on cells, but it blocks those sites rather than activating them, depressing the basal metabolic rate. The liver normally produces some RT3 when it is in the process of converting T4 to T3. Under periods of stress or illness, more RT3 is made than regular T3 as a way of conserving energy until the stress is relieved.

Elevated RT3 levels can be triggered by chronic stress (creating high levels of cortisol), adrenal fatigue, low ferritin levels (ferritin is your storage form of iron), restrictive diets, acute injury or illness, and chronic disease. As you'll read in the next chapter, these factors are the very same things that contribute to thyroid malfunction.

Endocrinologists generally do not recognize the importance of elevated RT3 levels or consider it an indicator of thyroid dysfunction.

Holistic doctors tend to disagree; they see elevated levels of RT3, even when TSH, free T3, and free T4 values are normal, as a reflection of a deeper thyroid problem at the cellular level. In the same research paper cited above, Kent Holtorf calls this a problem with "cellular hypothyroidism." According to Dr. Holtorf:

> Reverse T3 is actually an "antithyroid"—T3 is the active thyroid hormone that goes into the cells and stimulates energy and metabolism. Reverse T3 is a mirror image—it actually goes to the receptors and sticks there, and nothing happens. So it blocks the thyroid effect. Reverse T3 is kind of a hibernation hormone; in times of stress and chronic illness, it lowers your metabolism. So many people seemingly have normal thyroid hormone levels, but if they have high reverse T3, they're actually suffering from hypothyroidism.

This explains why many patients who are taking synthetic T4 medications (such as Oroxine, Synthroid, Levoxyl, et cetera) continue to suffer symptoms. The root of their problem is not that their bodies produce insufficient T4 but that some form of stress—inflammation, poor diet, toxicity, mental stress—is triggering their bodies to overproduce RT3. And addressing the root of the problem, as we'll learn in the next chapter, is the key to managing thyroid malfunction.

3

The Root Causes
of Thyroid Malfunction

We tend to think of thyroid malfunction as a modern malady exacerbated by the warp speed of the world we live in and the impurities we ingest. And while this is generally true, thyroid problems have haunted us for a long time.

The Chinese referred to thyroid illness in writings dating as far back as 2700 BCE. The seminal Ayurvedic textbook, the Sushruta Samhita, described hyperthyroidism, hypothyroidism, and goiter. The ancient Greeks bemoaned the horrors of Graves' disease long before it acquired that name, and during the mid-seventeenth century the thyroid was recognized as, well, the *thyroid;* its name derives from the Greek word for shield, as the gland looks somewhat like the shields early Greeks used in battle.

In modern times, our understanding of the thyroid gland has advanced, but we are still exploring all the intricacies of its function. What we have learned is that the thyroid gland is like a very delicate flower that needs to be watered daily and meticulously cared for. If there is any problem anywhere in the body, whether it comes from lack of nourishment, electromagnetic exposure, infections, or an overload of stress or toxins, this little flower will wilt, taking our physiology down with it. On the brighter side, if we give a little more attention to our bodies, resting, nourishing, and detoxifying them, our thyroid glands will bounce right back, giving us the glowing health and metabolism we long for.

THE ROOT OF ALL BALANCE: THE DOSHAS

Ayurveda prides itself on identifying imbalances at the deepest level. Before we unfold the numerous causes of thyroid dysfunction, it is imperative to understand that whatever the disease or symptoms may be—hair loss, arrhythmias, weight gain, fatigue, hyperthyroidism, hypothyroidism, Hashimoto's thyroiditis, Graves' disease, even thyroid cancer—we must first consider the balance of the three doshas. If you treat the symptoms without balancing the three doshas, your results will be minimal and temporary.

Chapter 1 describes the three doshas in detail. To briefly review:

- Vata: Represents the elements of space and air. Its qualities are quick, light, cold, dry, rough, subtle, mobile, erratic, and dispersing.
- Pitta: Represents the elements of fire and water. Its qualities are light, hot, oily, sharp, liquid, sour, and pungent.
- Kapha: Represents the elements of earth and water. Its qualities are heavy, cold, oily, slow, slimy, dense, soft, static, and sweet.

Vata: A Trigger for Thyroid Malfunction

When imbalanced, vata tends to emaciate the body's tissues, causing osteoporosis, weight loss, or thinning hair. Imbalanced vata moves thoughts quickly through the mind, so you absorb information quickly but then forget it quickly. Your physiology runs fast under the influence of vata, and you can become fatigued, especially if you force your body to keep up this level of hyperactivity day after day.

Have you noticed that many of these symptoms of vata imbalance are also characteristics of thyroid imbalance?

Throughout my thirty years of practice, I have seen hundreds of instances of vata types contributing to their thyroid problems by weakening their endocrine systems through incessant talking and boundless activity—which are on full display when they visit my office. This is a recipe for adrenal burnout and is the first step toward thyroid weakness. The endocrine glands cannot handle this amount of intense activity. The adrenals and thyroid glands are the batteries we run on. When depleted, they require a recharge, which is accomplished through proper rest, nourishing diet, and an early bedtime.

In the early stages, vata aggravation and hyperactivity can push the thyroid gland into a hyperthyroid (or overactive) state. But over time the gland will fatigue and become hypothyroid (or underactive) and unable to produce enough hormones.

Supporting the Thyroid by Balancing Vata

Vata aggravation can weaken not only the thyroid gland but the whole endocrine system, as well as the seven dhatus (tissues) and, as a result, the entire physiology that is nourished by those dhatus. Any treatments that you undertake for a thyroid condition will work more effectively if, at the same time, you learn to balance vata with the following practices:

Have a regular routine. Go to bed, wake up, and eat your meals at about the same time every day. The body and hormonal system work better when you follow established patterns for meals and bedtime.

Go to bed no later than 10:00 p.m. The hours before midnight are the most rejuvenative for sleeping. Go to bed when you feel the first impulse that you are tired. For some people this could be as early as 8:00 p.m., but it should not be later than 10:00 p.m. If you stay up later than that, you will get a second wind, which pushes your endocrine system to make more hormones at a time when the glands are fatigued and need rest, much like whipping a tired horse. You will be able to stay up, but the next day the fatigue will set in as your endocrine glands tank.

Do not rush through the day. Rushing around and multitasking will most certainly deplete your endocrine system. Vata types do need exercise, but since your physiology is figuratively running on a treadmill all day, vigorous exercise can also be a strain for your hormones. To support vata, it is best to favor gentle exercises such as walking, yoga, tai chi, stretching, and Pilates; avoid jogging.

Eat an unctuous diet. Lack of fat will throw vata out of balance very quickly, so fill your diet with unctuous foods like warm milk, ghee, olive oil, nuts, seeds, avocados, and soft curd cheeses, such as ricotta, fresh mozzarella, paneer, and cottage cheese. (Most of my patients avoid fat to a fault, disabling much of their endocrine system function and throwing vata more and more out of balance.)

Practice *abhyanga* (daily oil massages). If you have light skin, use olive or almond oil in the cooler months and coconut oil in the summer months; if you have darker skin, use sesame oil in the winter months and coconut oil in the summer. Apply the oil to your whole body, rubbing clockwise on the joints and downward on the long bones. Leave the oil on your body for at least 20 minutes; then you can shower it off, or leave it on if you prefer. Do this on a daily basis if you have the time and, if not, as many times during the week as you can manage. Keeping your body "unctuous" will further help in your attempts to keep this very dry dosha balanced in your body.

Eat warm, cooked foods. Avoid cold, light foods such as salads, which will aggravate vata. Also avoid raw foods, which constitute all the elements of vata: cold, dry, light, and rough.

Get outside. The elements outside in nature are the elements of kapha: earth and water. These are the antidotes to the spacey, drying elements of vata. Thus, it is imperative that vata types try to get outside as often as possible to infuse these elements into their physiology. Most people will tell you they feel calmer and sleep much better at night when they have been outdoors during the day, and that is due to the naturally kapha-supporting, vata-balancing influence of earth and water.

In the warmer months walk directly on the earth or the sand at the beach with your shoes off. Try to have direct contact with nature, as the electrons from the earth have a tremendous capability of grounding even the most spaced-out vata types. In fact, I recommend you read *Earthing: The Most Important Health Discovery Ever!* by Clinton Ober. He provides tremendous amounts of research and insight into the healing that is possible if we walk on the earth without shoes, as the rubber soles of shoes prevent the flow of this vital life energy up into our bodies.

Find peace and quiet. Vata types are sensitive to sounds. Minimize the time you spend with loud people, loud events, television, and so on, and point yourself toward peace and quiet. Take up prayer, meditation, or simply the solitude of nature to settle your active physiology.

Stay warm. Cold aggravates vata. Always dress properly in cold weather, and always cover your head, the location of a very important vata sub-dosha, prana vata, which governs our thoughts.

Using the Skin to Stay Balanced during the Vata Stage of Life

We are born in the kapha stage of life. This means that in the early childhood years the elements of kapha, earth and water, are more prevalent. This is why children tend to have frequent runny noses, coughs, and colds. Their body is making lubrication for the joints (shleshaka kapha; see page 28), and this lubrication can spill into the lungs and sinuses, for instance, in the form of phlegm.

The teen years into the twenties and thirties compose the pitta stage of life, when the elements of pitta, fire and water, become more pronounced in our physiology. As the liver, a pitta organ, automatically heats up, this heat can spread into the whole body, creating pitta-related problems, reflected on the skin as acne or in the temperament, such as flare-ups of anger. (Yes, even the ancient rishis stated in their texts to be patient with children in the teen years as they become irritable and moody!)

As we get older, into our forties and beyond, the element of vata takes over, creating drying of the joints, skin, mouth, vaginal tract, and other areas. Fears and anxieties can take hold as the vata in the mind (prana vata) becomes aggravated. Osteoporosis can set in as the bones become dry and brittle. Arthritis inflicts terrific pain as the joints lose their lubrication and dry up. The eyes and mouth can also dry up. Drying of the vaginal wall can occur, causing intercourse to be painful.

The ancient rishis of India said that the best way to combat vitiated vata and the accompanying dryness as we age is with daily oil massage. This is yet another example of their wisdom that we should heed.

Consider: Most holistic practitioners recommend that their patients take supplements of fish oils or other oils, such as primrose or flaxseed oil, for their omega-3 fatty acids and other nutrients. But they fail to take into account that these oils must travel through our digestive tract, particularly the liver and gallbladder. The liver has a difficult time digesting these concentrated sources of fats, and when they enter the gallbladder they increase the risk of formation of what is known as bile "sludge." Normally bile has a watery consistency; if too much fat infiltrates at one time and it becomes sludgy, it cannot flow properly and numerous problems can result (see chapter 7 for details). When I trained with Dr. Mishra, I often heard patients ask, "Should I take fish oil?" He would always say, "No! Eat the fish!"

The ancients were wise to note that these fats are good for our health when eaten in moderate amounts as part of our normal diet. But when we need larger amounts of oil, as we do in the later stages of our life to balance vata tendencies, instead of swallowing large amounts of oil all at once in supplement form, it would be better to apply them to the skin, allowing for absorption directly into the bloodstream, which avoids disruption of our digestive systems.

Keep in mind that the skin is the largest organ in the body; it releases toxins, and it can also take in almost everything applied onto it. Think of the skin as lots of little mouths—whatever you put on it goes directly into the bloodstream, more quickly than if you swallow it! This can be a bad thing if you put toxic skin-care products on your skin. On the plus side, however, many medications and even herbs can be taken transdermally (that is, through the skin).

In recent years research has shown that the skin possesses the capacity to generate several hormones and substances with hormone-like activity, and it is, in fact, being reclassified as an endocrine organ. These findings put a novel spin on our understanding of the skin's role in disorders of the human organism. Information has been rapidly accumulating over the past several years explaining the skin's role in endocrine-related functions, including the expression and function of specific hormone receptors, the synthesis of hormones, and the activation, inactivation, and elimination of the hormones in specialized cells of the skin.

Given that the skin is now thought to be integral to proper endocrine function, that most hormones are made from the components of fat, and thyroid health is dependent on the health of the rest of the endocrine system, it would greatly benefit your hormone levels and thyroid to give your skin the raw materials it needs to make hormones through the application of oils. This is especially true for women after menopause; it is estimated that the skin is responsible for the formation of 75 percent of the estrogens in women before menopause and for close to 100 percent of estrogens after menopause.

For those of us in the vata stage of life, oil massage on a regular basis, at least three to five times a week, helps keep the body properly lubricated, preventing vata from falling further out of balance and mitigating the anxieties and insomnia that can come with aging, not to mention the stiffness and joint pain.

There's Something Fishy about Fish Oil . . .

Fish oil is a phenomenon. Just ask its proponents. One of the most common supplements today, fish oils are loaded with omega-3s, which our bodies need but cannot produce; we must ingest them with our food. Omega-3s are thought to be crucial for the normal growth and development of the brain and the prevention of cardiovascular disease, some cancers, mood disorders, and, given their role in reducing inflammation, arthritis. Everyone is on the fish oil bandwagon: physicians, holistic practitioners, and nutritionists.

So while I hate to be the bearer of bad news, it turns out that fish oils are not as advertised. They can, counterintuitively, sometimes cause the very problems you seek to prevent with them.

Part of the problem results from the fact that most of the data on the benefits of omega-3s came from studies that looked at the consumption of fish, not fish oil supplements. Now that the studies are turning toward examinations of these supplements, the results are somewhat troublesome.

First, let me disabuse people of the notion that swallowing perles of oil at high doses, rather than eating foods rich in omega-3s, is a good idea. Consumption of fish oil strains the digestive system, especially the liver and gallbladder. And as we age, our ability to absorb oils decreases due to decreased production of the lipase enzyme by the pancreas.

Next, let's note that many of the fish oil supplements contain heavy metals due to poor purification processes, while others are rancid—that is, their fats are partially or completely oxidized. Light, oxygen exposure, and heat can all contribute to the oxidative process. This means that the oil has degraded because the oxygen in the air forms dangerous compounds full of free radicals that cause long-term harmful effects on your health, such as organ toxicity—especially to the liver, accelerated hardening of the arteries, and numerous other health conditions, such as cancer.

In 2016 the top three fish oil supplements in the United States were shown to have oxidation levels up to four times higher than recommended safe levels. And indeed, studies are now showing how both diabetes and cancer rates increased in those taking fish oils, including a threefold increase of melanoma and increased risks of prostate cancer and cancer in women. In addition, studies have now shown that the use of these supplements did not in fact reduce heart attacks, strokes, or deaths from heart disease, as had been hoped. And a 2010 study published in the *Journal of the American Medical Association* demonstrated that fish oil supplements taken during pregnancy have no effect on post-partum depression and do not help babies' brains develop more quickly. On the contrary, a 1992 article published by Wainwright et al. demonstrated that brain development is actually deterred by high doses of omega-3 fatty acids in fish oils.

It is probably best to conclude with the tried and true principles of diet—eat the fish, and don't assume that if a little of something is good for you, then more should be better. Fish, after all, provides more than just omega-3s. It also contains zinc, amino acids, and vitamin D, to name a few of its numerous nutrients. Isolating an "active" ingredient in a food—taking it out of context with nature, in much higher doses than the original food contained—is a practice taken out of the pharmaceutical playbook, which is bound to give side effects and toxicity.

DIETARY FACTORS PREVENTING THE CONVERSION OF T4 TO T3

As the last chapter described, proper thyroid function involves the conversion of T4 to T3, a process in which both the liver and the gut flora play a key role. In addition, the following nutrients are needed for this conversion to occur: iodine, iron, magnesium, selenium, zinc, and vitamins A, B_{12}, and D. Many people will be deficient in these nutrients at some point in their lives and therefore suffer disruptions to their thyroid function. To stave that off, pay attention to your diet and ensure that you are eating a variety of the foods that contain the nutrients you need to maintain a healthy thyroid.

Iodine

The body does not make iodine, so we must eat it in our diet. Don't take synthetic iodine—it is easy to overdose with it, and high levels of iodine can cause some of the same symptoms as iodine deficiency, including goiter, thyroid gland inflammation, and thyroid cancer. High levels of iodine can also reduce the synthesis of thyroid hormone and may even cause the thyroid gland to overproduce thyroid hormones, creating hyperthyroidism.

Foods high in iodine are cow's milk, cheese, seafood, eggs, saltwater fish, cranberries, and yogurt. Another good source is sea vegetables obtained from the Atlantic Coast, such as kombu (kelp), arame, hiziki, and wakame; try cooking with them once or twice a week or sprinkle your foods with a little granulated kelp a few times a week. Don't go overboard with kelp and seaweed, however, since they contain tremendous amounts of naturally occurring iodine.

Iron

Not only is iron needed for the conversion of T4 to T3, but low iron prevents normal thyroid function overall. This is because iron carries oxygen to all the cells of your body and the thyroid cannot work properly if deprived of adequate amounts of oxygen. Good sources of iron include medjool dates, raisins, prunes, dried apricots, Black Mission figs, cooked beets, blackstrap molasses, and cooked greens. It is common for iron to be low in a vegetarian diet; if you are a vegetarian, you must work extra hard at keeping your iron levels up.

If your iron levels are low and your doctor prescribes an iron supplement, you might want to consider taking an iron *bhasma*. According to the ancient rishis, the iron molecule (and also that of other minerals, such as zinc, calcium, and silica) was too large to enter the cells. They recommended burning the mineral repeatedly into an ash, with each incineration decreasing the size of the molecule until it became small enough (reaching the size of a nanoparticle) to enter the cells. The resultant mineral, known as a bhasma, is widely used in Ayurveda and is said to allow the adequate absorption of the mineral.

Magnesium

Magnesium not only stimulates the thyroid gland to produce T4 but also plays a role in converting T4 to T3. And at the same time it can prevent the overproduction of thyroid hormones, resulting in hyperthyroidism. Almost everyone in our country is magnesium deficient for a number of reasons: Our soil is depleted; the cortisol released from the adrenal glands under periods of stress flushes magnesium out of the body; and every pharmaceutical depletes the body's stores of magnesium. Other causes of magnesium deficiency are overconsumption of alcohol, excessive sugar intake, phosphates in soft drinks, the phytic acid found in the hulls of seeds and the bran of grains, and oxalates from foods such as raw green leafy vegetables (cooking the greens allows the oxalates to evaporate, making them safe for consumption), cocoa, and black tea; the tannic acid in tea binds magnesium and carries it out of the body. The lower our magnesium levels become, the more difficult it is to absorb iodine, which can affect thyroid function. Foods high in magnesium are cooked greens, wheat, almonds, cashews, molasses, buckwheat, pecans, walnuts, filberts, rye, coconut, figs, apricots, dates, collards, avocados, parsley, prunes, sunflower seeds, barley, raisins, and sweet potatoes.

Selenium

The conversion of T4 to T3 cannot take place without adequate selenium. In addition, some researchers suggest that after iodine, selenium is probably the next most important mineral affecting the thyroid's function, and in fact the thyroid contains more selenium by weight than any other organ. Both low and excessively high levels of iodine can disrupt thyroid function, and selenium can protect the thyroid from the damage caused by high iodine and also from any oxidative damage caused by the normal reactions that occur on a daily basis as the thyroid gland makes its hormones. Your body does not make selenium, so you must get it through your diet. Just two Brazil nuts a day is enough to meet the recommended daily allowance (RDA) of selenium. Other sources include yellowfin tuna, halibut, sardines, turkey, chicken, legumes, nuts, seeds, and eggs.

Zinc

Zinc is essential for the synthesis of thyroid hormones and, if low, may result in hypothyroidism. Conversely, low thyroid function can create a zinc deficiency as the thyroid hormones are needed for adequate absorption of zinc. Good sources of zinc include beans, nuts, chicken, oysters, whole grains, and dairy products. As in the case of iron, if you want to take a zinc supplement, consider a zinc bhasma to ensure proper absorption into the cells.

Vitamin A

Vitamin A is needed to activate thyroid hormone receptors, and low levels may depress thyroid function. In addition, if vitamin A levels are low the pituitary gland will increase its TSH production, which may cause swelling of the thyroid gland and at the same time reduce its uptake of iodine. However, researchers warn that not all hypothyroid patients should increase their intake of vitamin A supplements as high doses of vitamin A may actually decrease thyroid function. As usual, it is best to get your vitamins through your diet; just don't go overboard. Good sources of vitamin A include cooked carrots, yellow squash, sweet potatoes, cooked kale, dried apricots, butter, ghee, egg yolks, and whole milk.

Vitamin B$_{12}$

Forty percent of hypothyroid patients demonstrate a deficiency in vitamin B$_{12}$. Vitamin B$_{12}$ is found in animal proteins such as chicken, turkey, fish, lamb, milk and milk products, and eggs. B$_{12}$, is the only vitamin that is not found in a plant-based diet. B$_{12}$ is found in very small amounts in soil and plants, leading some vegans to think that they will be fine eating these foods for their only source of vitamin B$_{12}$. Some say certain foods such as spirulina, nori, nutritional yeast, tempeh, and barley grass are other nonanimal sources of B$_{12}$, and including these in the diet should be enough to prevent a B$_{12}$ deficiency. These claims have not proven to be true. The only way vegans, who eat no animal protein, can obtain adequate B$_{12}$ is to take B$_{12}$ supplements or eat cereals fortified with the vitamin. Ayurveda is not so keen on taking supplements since they are lacking prana, but instead try to convince their vegetarian patients to incorporate specific types of dairy products, as you will see in the upcoming chapters. If this is not an option for you, then you should be taking a B$_{12}$ supplement and eat foods fortified with B$_{12}$.

Vitamin D

The best way to ensure that you receive adequate vitamin D is sun exposure; as discussed earlier, absorption of UVB rays by the skin triggers the production of vitamin D. The problem is that most of us don't get out in the sun enough, or when we do, we use sunscreen.

You can get vitamin D through your diet but, again, for various reasons described throughout this book, I do not recommend foods fortified with synthetic versions of the vitamin. Instead, look for foods that naturally contain vitamin D. A three-ounce serving of mackerel or salmon will give you 90 percent of the RDA of vitamin D. Herring are another good choice; they have high levels of vitamin D because they thrive on plankton (a hearty source of vitamin D). Sardines are one of the best dietary sources of vitamin D; one small serving of sardines provides 101 percent of the RDA. Other good sources are tuna, trout, and catfish. One egg provides 21 percent of the RDA of vitamin D, and one cup of raw milk provides 24 percent. Vitamin D is also found in ghee.

During the winter months when you can't expose your skin to the sunlight we recommend the use of transdermal vitamin D, applied to the forearms in a thin layer twice a day. Later we will discuss in detail why oral supplementation of vitamin D is not recommended.

MALNUTRITION

The thyroid gland, like any gland or organ in the body, is dependent on a constant supply of nutrients. However, many of us suffer from lack of proper nourishment, inhibiting proper functioning of our bodies and minds.

You may ask, how could Americans be malnourished? We have more than enough food available to us, unlike our ancestors, who experienced long periods of starvation. In fact, the U.S. Centers for Disease Control reports that more than two-thirds (68.8 percent) of adults are considered overweight. More than one-third (35.7 percent) of adults are considered obese, and more than 1 in 20 (6.3 percent) have extreme obesity.

The industrialization of food and the advent of food processing account for this national health emergency. Many foods are stripped of their nutrients and loaded with chemicals to increase their shelf life. Many contain partially hydrogenated vegetable oils, which are similar to plastic in their chemical composition and cause serious clogging of the arteries. Artificial dyes have been shown to cause numerous cancers. Artificial sweeteners can burn the myelin sheath (the covering to the nerve tissue) and damage delicate brain and nerve tissue.

Industrial food production breaks basic laws of nature and makes a mockery of nutritional guidelines. As the ancient doctors of India counseled, to have value, all food should retain its pranic energy. It is this vibration that gives your cells the impulse to perform all their metabolic functions and the ability to communicate with each other. The more it is processed and the longer it sits on the shelf, the less nutritional value and pranic energy it retains. So any food that comes in a box, in a can, frozen, or otherwise processed and packaged for long life contains less "life energy" than fresh food and ultimately contributes to malnourishment.

Ayurveda concerns itself as well with the absorption of food—whether our body can break it down properly in the digestive tract and circulate it through our bloodstreams and cells. If our digestive process is weak, then full absorption will not occur. The adage, "You are what you eat" isn't exactly correct. Instead, we can say, "You are what you assimilate." For this reason, when I see new patients, one of the first things I assess and address is digestion.

We also have to take into consideration a patient's diet. Some foods are just too heavy to be taken up into the cells, like peanut butter and other nut butters, hard aged cheeses, red meats, soy products, chia seeds, hemp seeds, pumpkin seeds, mushrooms, winter squashes, and deep-fried foods. Because Americans have a penchant for eating these heavy channel-clogging foods, many people overcorrect and eat malnourishing diets in their attempts to lighten up their diets. Exhibit A is the ever-popular vegan diet.

The ancient doctors of India who wrote the textbooks on Ayurveda advised that we eat something from an animal at every meal. And this comes from a tradition of strict vegetarianism!

The rishis noted that you don't have to be vegetarian to maintain health. They did, however, say that if you are going to eat meat, limit it to the lighter meats that can gain entrance into your cells and not clog the delicate microchannels. These include chicken, turkey, fish, lamb, and rabbit. They even prescribed bone broth recipes to nourish extremely ill patients. As an alternative to or supplement to meat, they recommended dairy products like warm milk, yogurt, buttermilk, *takra* (another type of buttermilk), and fresh curd cheeses such as paneer, ricotta, mozzarella, cottage cheese, and farmer's cheese.

A vegan diet excludes all animal proteins, relying only on fruits, vegetables, grains, and beans. People on this diet can only exist for so long before their health deteriorates—the lack of protein, vitamin B_{12}, and calcium can lead, respectively, to hair loss, depression, and bone depletion.

Mara Kahn, author of *Vegan Betrayal: Love, Lies, and Hunger in a Plants-Only World,* notes, "There doesn't appear to be a single population of any significant size in the history of the world who survived on an exclusively plant-based diet." A journalist, she spent six years researching the history of vegetarianism. In her book she details the difference between a well-rounded vegetarian diet versus a depleting vegan diet. She writes, "Vegetarianism has a very long and noble history with verified health results. However, veganism . . . is a non-historical diet. . . . Its health benefits are not verified."

Not only are they not verified, but clinically I can attest to the fact that the hundreds of vegans I see are extremely ill and weak. Sometimes, after having subsisted on the heavy standard American diet for years, the transition to veganism gives them a newfound sense of lightness. However, once their stores of protein and B_{12} become depleted (usually within two years), their health starts to decline.

Even worse is a raw foods diet. My patients who have been eating a raw foods diet are even sicker than the vegans. This diet is too cold and light, aggravating vata dosha. Since vata imbalances can affect the mind, these patients can become spacey (vata is the element of space and air), depressed, hyper (if vata is too high, the mind moves too quickly), and anxious.

The argument for a raw foods diet is that cooking food kills the enzymes in food. What this argument fails to consider is cell absorption. You can't chew nearly enough to break down the fibers in raw vegetables so that you can absorb them; cooking the vegetables is required to soften the fibers and aid absorption. Adding spices enhances digestion, and the constituents of ghee (clarified butter) slide the food across the cell wall and into the cell. Remember, all the cell walls in your body are made of cholesterol, as is ghee, so ghee is an excellent vehicle to take the food into the cell, increasing absorption of nutrients and preventing malnutrition.

To reiterate, even though the cooking process may kill some of the enzymes, the net result is greater absorption than if the food is raw.

Chapter 8 will lay out proper diet in greater detail.

INFLAMMATION

Inflammation is another factor that prevents the conversion of T4 to T3, and it also inhibits the transport of T3 into the cells. I have read numerous health books, both mainstream and holistic, where inflammation is identified as the underlying cause of just about every disease. This is true; however, what almost everyone fails to discuss is what causes the inflammation and what to do about it.

Throughout my training with Dr. Mishra, one thing became increasingly clear: for optimum health, we must keep the liver functioning smoothly and maintain good growth of friendly bacteria in the gut. However, in our modern society, with our chronic overuse of pharmaceuticals and highly processed diet, the liver and gut are suffering, and as a result, they are at the root of the inflammation that triggers many of our ailments.

The liver carries out hundreds of functions in our bodies. Among many other things, it manages blood sugar; works more than any other organ to detoxify the body; secretes bile, which aids in the metabolism of fats, such as cholesterol and triglycerides; makes proteins for blood clotting; regulates our digestion; metabolizes hormones; and manufactures blood from the food we eat. It is the heaviest and largest internal organ in the human body.

Everything we swallow has to be scanned by the liver, since it is the liver's job to filter the blood coming from the digestive tract before it is distributed to the rest of the body. As a result, almost every American has some weakness in the liver due to the highly processed diet we've been raised on and the overuse of pharmaceuticals. Jeff Hays's documentary film, *Doctored,* explains that while Americans compose only 5 percent of the world's population, we consume an incredible 50 percent of all pharmaceutical drugs. This combination of a diet filled with chemicals and overuse of pharmaceuticals has created enormous toxicity and overburdened the liver.

When the liver is overwhelmed with acid toxins, it will eventually overheat. This overheating becomes a huge source of inflammation: since the liver makes blood from the food we eat, the blood starts to overheat as well. As this hot blood circulates, the entire body can suffer the consequences of this heat. In this way liver toxicity becomes the initial source of chronic inflammation, which creates the foundation for many diseases.

This is an extremely important point to understand, because modern medicine only monitors liver function through blood work, looking to see if there are elevated levels of the liver enzymes AST (or SGOT) and ALT (or SGPT). These enzymes are normally predominantly contained within liver cells and to a lesser degree in the muscle cells. If the liver is injured or damaged, these enzymes spill into the blood, raising the AST and ALT blood levels and signaling full-fledged liver disease.

However, these enzyme levels become elevated only once liver damage has become serious. The most effective time to intervene is long before that happens, when the liver is simply overloaded with toxins and overheated. An Ayurvedic practitioner uses pulse diagnosis to make this assessment. We begin treatment whenever we find any problems in the liver pulse (ranjaka pitta).

The second source of chronic inflammation in the body is a lack of friendly bacteria in the gut. These friendly bacteria are delicate and can easily be killed by too much stress, acidic digestive juices, and numerous drugs such as antibiotics, birth control pills, antacids, NSAIDs, and steroids. Once these beneficial bacteria die off, pathogenic microorganisms can move in and flourish in the gut.

This state of infection in the gut, whether caused by *Candida albicans* (the most common and widespread infection), small intestinal bacterial overgrowth (SIBO), parasites, or other bacteria, creates inflammation as a by-product of the immune system's assault on the pathogens.

Both acidic toxins in the liver and infection in the gut create the conditions for systemic inflammation. And it is this inflammation that can prevent the conversion of T4 into T3 and the entrance of T3 into the cells. See the section, "The Three Parts of the Immune System," chapter 5, page 97, for more on how to care for the liver and the gut.

....

ProTren: My Favorite Probiotic

Almost everyone knows now the important role that friendly bacteria play in a person's health. However, what most people do not know is that most of the probiotic cultures on the market are ineffective. In the early years of my practice I would instruct patients to get a good probiotic from their local health food store to treat their dysbiosis (a gut infection stemming from lack of friendly bacteria). In almost every case, though, the infection persisted. I found the same results when patients were eating good-quality probiotic yogurts or making their own yogurt.

Then a turning point occurred in my practice in 1992. I attended a seminar where a doctor from Europe spent several days showing us commercial probiotic cultures under a very expensive microscope. We were astonished to find that the cultures in every company's product were deficient. Only one company met the test: ProTren Intelligent Probiotics. When I contacted the company, they told me that it is quite difficult to process a probiotic without destroying the active cultures and that unless the company displays the words "100% potency guaranteed" on its product label, chances are that many of the live cultures will have died during processing.

Since I started recommending ProTren probiotics, it has been fairly easy for my patients to overcome chronic gut infections. For example, *Candida albicans* yeast overgrowth, which normally took a year or two to eradicate, now takes two months.

Dr. Mishra and I also experimented with various yogurt cultures, trying to make yogurt according to the strict Ayurvedic standards for use as a probiotic. The ancient doctors said that yogurt shouldn't taste too sour because the acidity could destroy the friendly bacteria. We tried several brands from various health food stores, but none of them lived up to these standards. We then tried making yogurt with various starters, but again without success.

However, when we used ProTren's yogurt starter, we found what we were looking for. The yogurt was the kind recommended in the ancient texts: very alkaline tasting and filled with the life essence of the friendly bacteria cultures. To this day I sell this yogurt starter in our office. I instruct my patients who use it to make probiotic yogurt to eat it at lunch only, when digestion is at its peak, since cold dairy is very mucous forming. I also teach them how to make drinks from the yogurt, including a medicinal lassi: combine $1/4$ cup of homemade yogurt with $3/4$ cup water, add a pinch of ground cumin and a few fresh cilantro leaves, blend well, and sip between bites of food. I also recommend hanging the yogurt in cheesecloth and letting it drip into a bowl overnight in the refrigerator and drinking this whey from the yogurt at lunch.

There may now be other companies that can guarantee their active probiotic cultures, but to be on the safe side, I continue to use ProTren, since I know for sure that it works.

TOXICITY

Ayurveda delineates four types of toxins:

- *Ama,* which comes from improper digestion of food and malabsorption into cells
- *Ama visha,* which arises from ama fermenting in our channels
- *Gara visha,* which comes from environmental xenobiotics accumulating in the body
- *Indravajraabhijanya visha,* which comes from electromagnetic radiation

The thyroid gland is sensitive to them all.

We teach our patients specific methods for removing each type of toxin (see below). I will not discuss the stronger detox protocols in this book, such as how to perform panchakarma (the premier Ayurvedic cleanse) at home, since it is important that patients be monitored by their doctors to make sure they are properly implementing their detox protocols, which are different for each patient. Cleansing on your own, without sufficient knowledge of the detox process, may ultimately backfire, especially if you pull out the toxins too quickly or haphazardly. This can result in rupture of the delicate microchannels of the body, which have to carry the toxins from the deeper tissues out through channels into bowel movements, urine, and sweat.

We do not recommend detoxification for children, as they are in the stage of life where they are building up their bodies and need more nourishment and nurturing. We also do not recommended detoxification for women who are pregnant or nursing, as the toxins can travel into the bloodstream and breast milk, adversely affecting the baby.

Ama

All the digestive organs (stomach, liver, gallbladder, pancreas) create what is called our "digestive fire"—the energy and mechanisms by which food is transformed and "cooked" once it comes into the digestive tract.

If your flame is too low (which can be detected in your pulse), it will be hard to digest the food, and ama can even form from healthy food. And some foods are just too dense or heavy to digest and assimilate well. Foods in this category would be cold milk, ice cream and frozen yogurt, hard aged cheeses, unfermented soy products (tofu, edamame, soy milk), beef and other red meats, pork, ham, sausage, bacon, hot dogs, processed lunch meats, and nut butters (peanut butter, almond butter, sunflower butter). If we eat food that is heavy at a time when our digestive fire is winding down, we do not digest it very well. Our internal flame mimics the sun: In the morning our digestive fire begins to ignite. By the middle of the day, when the sun is at its highest in the sky, our digestive fire is at its peak and most capable of digesting and assimilating foods. As the sun goes down, our digestive flame subsides as well. (And this is why it is best not to eat heavy foods early or late in the day.)

When food gets bogged down in our digestive "channel," as the ancient doctors called the large tube—the esophagus, stomach, and small and large intestines—that carries food after we swallow it, ama forms. Whether due to weak digestion or heavy food, ama causes malabsorption of nutrients into cells. As ama sits in the digestive channel, clogging it, it can lead to subsequent channels also becoming clogged, such as the sinuses or the ear canals, and it can breed infection. When you blow your nose or cough up mucus, you are looking at ama mixed in with the mucus.

One way to tell if you have made ama from the food you just ate is if you feel tired after eating. Other good indicators are stiffness in the body, sluggishness, and even depression as ama clogs and prevents the normal flow of fluids throughout the body. And finally, a white coating on the tongue indicates that you are producing ama from your food.

Ama is a cold toxin, and to clear it, we generally use heating treatments like hot tea with honey and warming spices such as ginger and black pepper. There are many recipes for clearing ama from the channels. Here is one of my favorites—it's a good recipe to make when you feel dense, heavy, weighed down, sluggish, stiff, and achy.

৩৭ *Tea to Detoxify Ama*

> Boil 1 quart of water for 5 minutes, and then pour the hot water into a stainless-steel insulated thermos. Add 2 green cardamom pods, 2 thin slices of ginger root, 2 black peppercorns, 1 whole allspice berry, 1 clove, and a $1/2$-inch piece of cinnamon stick. Seal the thermos, and let the spices steep for 20 minutes. Then start sipping slowly, drinking as much as you like at a time, for the next 4 hours. After 4 hours, the herbs will lose their effectiveness.

Ama Visha

When ama is stuck in our digestive channel, it starts to ferment and becomes ama visha. *Visha* means "poison"; ama visha is much more dangerous than ama, since it is now acidic and can penetrate deeply into the body, creating skin rashes, inflammation, autoimmune diseases, and cancer.

Ama visha is a very hot toxin, so it has to be pulled out using cooling spices and herbs. Here is one recipe.

৩৭ *Tea to Detoxify Ama Visha*

> Boil 1 quart of water for 5 minutes, and then pour the hot water into a stainless-steel insulated thermos. Add $1/2$ teaspoon of whole coriander seeds, $1/2$ teaspoon of slippery elm bark, and $1/4$ teaspoon of deglycerized licorice root (DGL). Seal the thermos, and let steep for 20 minutes; then sip slowly over the next 4 hours.

The coriander seed in this tea will pull out the ama visha and direct it to the urine and away from the skin. The slippery elm and DGL will lubricate the channels so that they don't rupture or become inflamed as this hot toxin is released. If you pull ama visha out too abruptly without directing it into bowel movements and urine, it can cause a rash on the skin, especially if you are using heating herbs and spices (ginger, pepper, cayenne) to pull it out. I have had several patients with an overload of ama visha do the classic maple syrup/cayenne pepper cleanse to try to remove it. As you can imagine, this cleanse is very heating and caused their whole body to break out in an itchy weeping rash that took several weeks to resolve.

Gara Visha

Whereas ama and ama visha are formed from the improper combustion of food inside the body, gara visha, the third type of toxin, comes from environmental xenobiotics such as air pollution, pesticides, pharmaceuticals and nutraceuticals, artificial sweeteners, additives and preservatives in our food, and synthetic skin-care products we put on our bodies. These toxins can make their way to deep levels of the body, including the bone marrow, triggering autoimmune diseases and cancer.

Gara visha has a hot acidic nature, so like ama visha, it can cause rashes on the skin as it exits through the sweat pores, so we have to be very careful when pulling it out, since it can rupture the physical channels on its way out through the bowel movements, urine, and sweat. The tea recipe below is a good way to detoxify gara visha. The herbs in the recipe are gentle on the liver, direct the toxins away from the skin, and lubricate the channels that carry them out.

ॐ Tea to Detoxify Gara Visha

Boil 1 quart of water for 5 minutes, and then pour the hot water into a stainless-steel insulated thermos. Add $^1/_4$ teaspoon of dried basil leaf (or 3 fresh basil leaves, torn), $^1/_4$ teaspoon of whole coriander seeds, $^1/_4$ teaspoon of guduchi, $^1/_4$ teaspoon of marshmallow root, $^1/_4$ teaspoon of neem leaf, $^1/_4$ teaspoon of dried mint (or 3 fresh mint leaves, torn), $^1/_4$ teaspoon of Indian sarsaparilla root, $^1/_4$ teaspoon of slippery elm bark, and 2 organic rosebuds.

In this tea, the guduchi pulls toxins from bone marrow and deep tissues (see page 109 for more on this herb). Coriander is used to direct these very hot toxins into the urine; Indian sarsaparilla root cleanses fatty tissues (where nasty chemicals are stored), neem leaf is used to purify the liver and the blood, and marshmallow root and slippery elm protect and lubricate the channels to prevent their rupture as these very hot toxins exit. The rosebuds are used to keep the formula cool.

Fluoride and the Thyroid

Fluoride is a by-product of the aluminum and fertilizer industries that is sold to American cities to fluoridate their water supply. It is a potent neurotoxin that can have devastating effects on the thyroid and, among other things, has been shown to decrease IQs in children.

In the 1930s, fluoride was used as a medication to manage an overactive thyroid. Fluoride displaces iodine in the thyroid gland, thereby decreasing the production of thyroid hormones. Its effects were so powerful that many patients suffered complete loss of thyroid function and had to discontinue treatment.

Despite the numerous published articles demonstrating fluoride's detrimental effects, the United States continues to add fluoride to municipal water supplies reaching 211 million Americans, or more than 67 percent of Americans, and about 6 million people receive fluoridated water in the United Kingdom. British researchers feel that 15,000 people may become afflicted with hypothyroidism in the UK as a result. Numerous countries have stopped fluoridating their water, including Germany, Sweden, Japan, the Netherlands, Finland, and Israel.

In 1958, Drs. Galetti and Joyet published a study in the *Journal of Clinical Endocrinology and Metabolism* demonstrating how fluoride can slow thyroid function. The patients in their study were given 2 milligrams of fluoride a day, which proved enough to decrease their thyroid activity. Today, in comparison, if you drink fluoridated tap water, you are taking in more than 6 milligrams of fluoride per day! It's little wonder that many people point to the use of fluoridated water as a contributing factor to the recent epidemic of hypothyroidism.

Fifty percent of the fluoride you ingest accumulates in your fat cells, slowly disrupting the normal biochemical reactions in your body and causing abnormal changes in your body's proteins. This in turn causes your immune system to produce antibodies to destroy these abnormal proteins, which can ultimately lead to an autoimmune reaction in the thyroid gland—either Hashimoto's thyroiditis or Graves' disease. Hashimoto's causes an underactive thyroid, or hypothyroidism, and Grave's causes an overactive thyroid condition, or hyperthyroidism.

Recent research linking fluoridated water consumption to thyroid problems has been well documented. It is directly or indirectly responsible for damaging thyroid gland cells, disrupting the conversion of T4 to T3, and mimicking TSH. It can also prevent the uptake of thyroid hormones at the receptor sites in all of the body's cells and prevent the production of TSH from the pituitary gland (remember, it is TSH, or thyroid-stimulating hormone, that gives the thyroid gland the signal to make more of its hormones).

Thyroid disease has skyrocketed over the past two decades, with an increase in 75 percent in neonatal hypothyroidism, now affecting 1 in every 2,370 births. Similar statistics hold true for the older populations.

Fluoride may be found in tap water, toothpaste, pesticides used in farming, dental products, and numerous other household products. Therefore, make sure your drinking water, toothpaste, and other household products are free of fluoride, and buy organic food as much as you can.

Heavy Metals

The thyroid gland is sensitive to any and all toxins. However, mercury, a heavy metal, is especially problematic because it is very similar in structure to iodine, which the thyroid gland needs to make hormones. If your thyroid gland makes the mistake of absorbing mercury instead of iodine, it won't be able to produce enough of its hormones, and the mercury in the thyroid could potentially cause an autoimmune reaction, because mercury is one of the deadliest chemical toxins known to mankind.

In addition, mercury is considered an extremely hot toxin, piercing through all seven tissues immediately as it enters the body and settling in the bone marrow, disrupting function there. It is actually quite easy to feel this disturbance in the pulse of a patient who is experiencing mercury toxicity.

Current chelation therapies used in conventional medicine for the removal of heavy metals like mercury from the blood include IV injections of EDTA (ethylenediaminetetraacetic acid), an amino acid. Another common chelating agent currently in use is DMPS (2,3-dimercapto-1-propanesulfonic acid). Since both are synthetically made, they themselves have toxic effects, the most common being a burning sensation at the site of injection, fever, headache, nausea, and vomiting. There is also the potential for life-threatening heart failure, a sudden drop in blood pressure, abnormally low blood levels of calcium, permanent kidney damage, and bone marrow depression.

Ayurveda uses fresh cilantro leaves for chelation of mercury and other heavy metals without all the side effects and toxicity of the synthetic chelating agents. There are numerous studies demonstrating cilantro's effectiveness in pulling out these highly toxic compounds.

In fact, cilantro is so potent at pulling out heavy metals that you need just a few tablespoons a day, eaten fresh, for a powerful effect. If you are using cilantro for detox, make sure you eat foods that bind the heavy metals you are chelating, leading them into bowel movements. Good binders are okra, taro root, arrowroot, and barley. Also eat white daikon radish and asparagus to direct the toxins into the kidneys. The gara visha detoxification tea on page 67 will also be helpful in releasing toxins in a safe manner.

Indravajraabhijanya Visha

Indravajraabhijanya visha, the fourth type of toxin, comes from electromagnetic frequencies (EMFs) and radiation emitted by such things as cell phones, computers, X-rays, cell phone towers, and Wi-Fi. As previously mentioned, EMFs mix with prana and are delivered to all the organs, glands, and systems through the vibrational channels. Since it is the prana that gives cells their intelligence to perform all of their functions, this type of toxin can cause cancer as the cellular functions become disrupted. In fact, it is well known that electromagnetic radiation is a common cause of thyroid cancer.

The natural world is itself the best remedy for and barrier against EMF toxicity. Here are several tips for people who are exposed to this type of radiation on a daily basis:

- Lie directly on the sand at the beach for one half hour whenever you can. The sand will absorb the EMFs from your body.

- Walk directly on the earth in your bare feet.
- Sit up against trees, as their bark can pull radiation out of your body.
- Walk in the moonlight.
- Basil is commonly used to pull out electromagnetic radiation. Try tearing up to three fresh basil leaves and putting them in your drinking water to sip on throughout the day. Or put a handful of fresh basil leaves in a tub of warm water and soak in it for twenty minutes three times a week.
- Put plants around your computer to absorb some of the EMFs.
- Get out in nature, where the prana is pure, as much as you can.

Six Vegetables Used for Detox

In Ayurveda, six vegetables are commonly eaten for detoxification: white daikon radish and asparagus, which cleanse the kidneys; loki squash and bitter gourd (also known as karela or bitter melon), which cleanse the liver; and taro root and okra, which bind toxins and direct them into bowel movements.

- **White daikon radish:** It looks like a carrot but is larger; peel and chop like a carrot for cooking.
- **Asparagus:** This is the same asparagus you'll find in conventional grocery stores.
- **Loki squash:** Available at Asian or Indian markets; peel and chop into one-inch chunks for cooking.
- **Bitter gourd/bitter melon/karela:** Available at Indian markets; slice into rounds, cook, then discard the large inner seeds; eat the skin.
- **Taro root:** Looks like an oblong coconut on the outside; peel and chop like a potato for cooking.
- **Okra:** You can find this in many conventional grocery stores these days. Slice into thin rounds.

You can add all six of these vegetables to a split mung dahl lentil soup called *kitcheree*. Split mung dahl is basically the green mung bean, which has had its hard outer shell removed and been cut in half for easy digestion and assimilation. Try to find organic split mung dahl for best results. You can prepare this lentil soup three or more times a week, depending on how sluggish, fatigued, and stiff you feel (all signs of toxicity). There are hundreds of recipes for kitcheree. Here is a common one for detoxification.

ॐ Kitcheree for Detoxification

One cup of detoxifying vegetables (from the list above), roughly chopped

2–3 handfuls organic split mung dahl

2–3 handfuls organic white basmati rice (optional)

1 teaspoon ghee

3 pinches salt

2 pinches ground coriander

2 pinches ground cumin

2 pinches ground fennel

2 pinches ground turmeric

Freshly ground black pepper, to taste

Combine all the ingredients in a medium pot, and add enough water to cover by about 1 inch. Bring to a boil, then reduce the heat and let simmer until the lentils are soft and the vegetables are cooked through, 20 to 25 minutes, stirring occasionally. Check periodically to see if more water is needed. You can make it as thick or as thin as you like.

IS SOY A TRIGGER FOR THYROID MALFUNCTION?

The battle over whether soy products can adversely affect the thyroid gland continues. Soy products such as tofu, soy milk, and edamame contain estrogen-like compounds called isoflavones. Proponents of soy recommend it for reducing menopausal symptoms, preventing cancer and heart disease, and weight loss, among other things. On the other side of the debate are those who believe soy is an endocrine disruptor that affects normal thyroid function, promotes the growth of some types of cancer, impairs female fertility, depresses growth in children, and causes fatty deposits in the liver.

Part of the controversy lies in the fact that soy has different properties depending on whether it is fermented. Soybeans and their products have enzyme inhibitors that block the digestion of protein, which can cause numerous health problems. Soybeans also contain hemagglutinin, which causes red blood cells to clump together. Fermenting the soy deactivates the enzyme inhibitors and the hemagglutinin. So fermented soy products like tempeh, miso, soy sauce, and tamari are generally safe to eat, but unfermented soy is a definite health problem and a trigger for thyroid malfunction.

My teacher, Dr. Mishra, could tell when a patient was eating a lot of unfermented soy because he would detect severe clogging of the pulse, which he termed a "tofu pulse." He immediately instructed those patients to discontinue consuming soy products, and as time went by, the stickiness in their blood went away.

I will present the research here, but clinically I can also share with you what I see on a daily basis in my Ayurvedic practice. Research is good, and I have cited research throughout this book to support my work. But you can't discount patterns that emerge as you see thousands of patients over months and years. Experience matters. And I can emphatically say this: Soy has a definite anti-thyroid effect. It slows thyroid function and triggers thyroid disease—even more so than the touted goiter-producing foods such as the cruciferous vegetables (cauliflower, broccoli, cabbage, brussels sprouts, and kale).

On numerous occasions when I have found clinical or subclinical hypothyroidism lurking in a patient's pulse, I performed an experiment. I asked the patient if he was consuming soy, and if he was, I had him discontinue it for a month and then return for a second evaluation. In many cases, the thyroid gland was no longer problematic on the second visit, and the patient required no treatment for whatever problem had brought him to my office.

This was especially true in cases of both mild and severe arrhythmias of the heart. I've had patients with arrhythmia whose pulse revealed thyroid malfunction, and when they stopped using soy products like soy milk and tofu daily, their heart rhythms miraculously returned to normal. Some of these patients were on beta-blockers and other medications to restore their heart rhythm but had been unsuccessful in that effort because they weren't getting to the root of the problem: soy consumption triggering thyroid malfunction.

I know that some of you will demand research to buttress my case, so here it is. Let's start with researchers Daniel Doerge and Daniel Sheehan, two of the Food and Drug Administration's (FDA) experts on soy. Here is an excerpt from a letter they wrote protesting the positive health claims for soy issued by the FDA:

> There is abundant evidence that some of the isoflavones found in soy, including genistein and equol, a metabolite of daidzein, demonstrate toxicity in estrogen sensitive tissues and in the thyroid. This is true for a number of species, including humans. Additionally, isoflavones are inhibitors of the thyroid peroxidase which makes T3 and T4, and can generate thyroid abnormalities, including goiter and autoimmune thyroiditis. There exists a significant body of animal data that demonstrates goitrogenic and even carcinogenic effects of soy products. Moreover, there are significant reports of goitrogenic effects from soy consumption in human infants and adults.

In addition, studies have found that children with autoimmune thyroid disease are more likely to have been fed soy-based infant formula. This was the culprit in the case of Elizabeth and Megan, whose case history was presented in the preface to this book. In fact, there has been so much research to support this claim that Dr. Mike Fitzpatrick, an internationally known toxicologist who has extensively researched the issue of soy formulas and their impact on thyroid function, is calling for soy formula manufacturers to remove the isoflavones, "the agents that are most active against the thyroid," from their products. He also warns against the adult consumption of soy products and states that "people with hypothyroidism should seriously consider avoiding soy products," noting that failure to do so will ultimately result in an increase in thyroid disorders.

The French Center for Cancer Research issued a warning that soy products should not be eaten by children under three years of age or by women who have breast cancer or are at risk of the disease. The Israeli Health Ministry suggests that soy consumption be limited in young children and avoided altogether in infants.

In *The Whole Soy Story*, author Kaayla Daniels, Ph.D., notes that consuming more than 30 mg of soy isoflavones per day has a toxic effect on the thyroid gland. The traditional Asian diet, which we may tend to think of as being soy heavy, actually ranges from just 10 to 30 mg of isoflavones per day, mostly from soybeans that have not been industrially processed or genetically modified. However, in the United States, people take in 80 to 100 mg of isoflavones a day by consuming soy milk, soy nuts, soy protein shakes, foods enriched with soy, and soy-based supplements, sometimes adding up to a whopping 300 mg a day of isoflavones. More than 90 percent of the soy consumed in the United States is genetically modified. In addition, soybeans are one of our most pesticide-contaminated foods.

Since many people eat soy to boost their estrogen levels, I would caution: Many thyroid patients have a problem with a high estrogen/low progesterone ratio (for reasons outlined later this book). High estrogen levels can cause growths, such as thyroid nodules, fibroid tumors, and cysts on the breasts and ovaries. Soy is highly estrogenic, so for these people, it is best to avoid soy altogether. If you want to boost your reproductive hormones for relief of hot flashes, insomnia, emotional upset, or the other problems that low hormones can bring, always do it in a manner that maintains the balance between estrogen and progesterone. There are numerous herbs that can be taken to maintain this delicate balance (see page 148 for some examples). I myself am reluctant to use even the Ayurvedic herbs that increase estrogen, such as shatavari, unless I have balanced the thyroid hormones and can keep the levels of progesterone normal.

A study published in *Cancer Research* in 2001 demonstrated that soy isoflavones even at low concentrations can stimulate breast tumor growth and antagonize the antitumor effects of tamoxifen (an antiestrogenic medication used in estrogen-sensitive breast cancer patients). The authors cautioned women with current or past breast cancer to be aware of the risks of potential tumor growth that can occur if you are consuming soy products.

PROLONGED
ADRENAL STRESS

The adrenal glands are called on during periods of stress to produce hormones such as adrenaline and cortisol, which create the "fight or flight" response. So many bodily functions, such as digestion, shut down when we experience danger. If this stress response is just occasional, then the body will recalibrate itself after the stressful situation passes. However, many of us live in a state of constant fight or flight, with too many stressors creating continual release of cortisol, leaving the endocrine system imbalanced. Prolonged cortisol elevation decreases the liver's ability to clear excess estrogens from the blood. Excess estrogen increases levels of thyroid-binding globulin (the proteins that bind to thyroid hormone in order to transport it through the body). When thyroid hormone is bound to TBG, it is inactive, causing less available thyroid hormone to be used by the cells.

High cortisol levels also reduce the conversion of T4 to T3. Thus, adrenal imbalance can cause hypothyroid symptoms without problems in the thyroid gland itself. In such cases, treating the thyroid is both unnecessary and ineffective. Addressing the adrenals is the key to improving thyroid function. (We'll discuss how to support the adrenals in the next chapter.)

BLOOD WORK
TO EVALUATE THYROID FUNCTION

When undergoing testing for thyroid function, always assess TSH, free T4, free T3, RT3, and thyroid antibodies—thyroid peroxidase antibodies (TPOAb) and thyroglobulin antibodies (TgAb). The latter are antibodies produced by your immune system that would be elevated in cases of autoimmune disease of the thyroid gland.

Always keep in mind, however, that because the thyroid gland has effects on every cell of your body, and the cells of your body are in a constant state of flux, thyroid function tests may change as the stressors on your body come and go. For example, TSH might be elevated if you had a recent illness, or your RT3 could be elevated if you are on a restrictive vegan diet. Or maybe the blood work will appear normal even though you are symptomatic. Remember, the thyroid gland has to go through a few stages of weakness before that weakness will be reflected in your blood work. But you can experience a wide range of thyroid symptoms even when the thyroid is in its earliest stages of decline. As we have discussed, the idea is to fix the root of the problem—the reason for the weakness—as soon as possible, before it becomes obvious on blood work or develops into full-blown thyroid disease.

4

Thyroid and
Adrenal Interactions

The glands of the endocrine system coordinate a wide range of bodily functions and work on our behalf to regulate numerous internal processes that may be taken for granted until the system weakens and subsequently fails us. The functions of these various glands may fluctuate throughout your life, rising and falling with the stressors and challenges you encounter. But don't automatically resort to pharmaceutical treatment without first attempting to balance, heal, and support your glandular system. If you give your body proper rest, nourishment, and good-quality herbs, you will be amazed to find that it can actually heal itself. Identifying and addressing the various causes of endocrine gland burnout and working on eliminating those causes and supporting the glands back to their normal function is the true art of practicing medicine.

All the glands of the endocrine system work in concert, with a weakness in one ultimately affecting another. However, here we are going to pay specific attention to interactions between the thyroid and adrenal glands. Both produce hormones that affect your energy levels, and when weak, both glands produce similar symptoms, such as fatigue, forgetfulness, and depression. In addition, both glands become weakened from prolonged physical and mental stress. In fact, many people suffer from adrenal exhaustion, which leads to thyroid malfunction. They are then put on thyroid medication, but the fatigue continues since the adrenal glands are still weak. The root of the problem hasn't been addressed. Eventually both glands go through a period of hyperactivity to meet the demands of prolonged stress until they become exhausted, leading to hypothyroidism and hypo-adrenia, or low-functioning thyroid and adrenals. Fortunately most of the therapies in this book directed toward healing your thyroid gland will also strengthen the adrenal glands.

The adrenal glands release stress hormones, such as cortisol and adrenaline in response to a stressor. However, if the stress continues for long periods of time, without breaks in between, the adrenal glands can no longer meet the demands for a continuous supply of stress hormones, leaving them (and you) exhausted. These continual high levels of adrenal stress hormones disrupt the normal functions of the thyroid gland. Here are some of the reasons:

- Prolonged cortisol release caused by chronic stress prevents the liver from clearing excess estrogens from the blood. This excess estrogen increases the levels of thyroid TBG (thyroid binding globulin), the protein that the thyroid hormone attaches to as it is carried around the body to its final destination. If there is too much TBG circulating around, the thyroid hormone will remain inactive as thyroid hormone must be released from TBG to allow it to enter the cell to have its effect.
- High levels of cortisol decrease TSH, lowering thyroid hormone production.
- Cortisol inhibits the conversion of T4 to T3 and increases the conversion to T4 to reverse T3.
- Cortisol flushes magnesium out of the body, which is used for the conversion of T4 to T3. As magnesium levels drop, you become more anxious and hyper, further weakening both the thyroid and adrenal glands.
- Once the adrenal glands are exhausted and the cortisol levels are very low, the cell receptors do not respond to T3.

- Low adrenal function causes inflammation. Here are several ways inflammation can disrupt thyroid function:

  1. Immune system cells release cytokines (such as C-reactive protein, interleukin-6, and tumor necrosis factor alpha), which stimulate the movement of cells toward areas of inflammation, infection, and trauma. These cytokines have been known to cause hypothyroidism.

  2. Inflammation (resulting from adrenal exhaustion) depresses thyroid receptor site sensitivity, so even if your thyroid is producing its hormones (which look normal on blood work) they can't gain access to the inside of the cells.

  3. Inflammation can interfere with the proper transportation of iodine into your thyroid gland.

  4. Inflammation can decrease serotonin (a neurotransmitter that makes you feel happy and helps you focus), which then inhibits formation of TSH. When inflammation is present, the body uses your serotonin to make inflammatory proteins, thus depleting it.

As we try to restore balance to our endocrine system, we miss the big picture if we focus exclusively on just these glands or just this system. The body was compartmentalized solely to make it easy for doctors to study and learn, but this is a limited view of the way the body truly functions. Ayurveda prides itself on identifying the root causes, which are usually numerous and specific for each person, understanding that these root causes are usually far removed from where the symptoms are occurring.

SYMPTOMS OF THYROID WEAKNESS

When the thyroid gland is not functioning up to par, even if the blood work appears normal, it can have a range of effects in the body:

Bone loss: T3 provides the bone-building cells (called osteoblasts) with the fuel they need to manufacture bone. T3 also stimulates the production of alkaline phosphatase, an enzyme produced in the liver that is crucial to bone mineralization. Without enough T3, the process of breaking down the bones can occur more rapidly than the bones can be built up, resulting in decreased bone density and osteopenia or osteoporosis. There are numerous other reasons our bones can break down quickly when thyroid function is off, especially if vata is disturbed, because vata disturbances can break down any of the seven tissues, including bone.

Loss of hair, dry or brittle hair, and brittle nails: The ancient texts of Ayurveda say that the hair and nails are considered malas (roughly interpreted as "waste products") of the bones. Thus, hair falling out (including loss or thinning of eyebrows and eyelashes) and brittle nails are indications of weak bones and potentially of a thyroid imbalance. In addition, hair growth is dependent on the health of the thyroid gland since T3 and T4 regulate hair growth. Hair loss occurs when an enzyme converts testosterone to DHT (dihydrotestosterone). DHT attacks the hair follicles causing shrinkage until the follicles disappear completely, causing the hair to become finer, stop growing, and fall out. When the thyroid is hyper or hypo, testosterone converts to DHT at a much quicker rate. Fortunately, once the thyroid problem stabilizes, the hair loss tends to be reversible in most cases. Also take note: low iron levels are important for both normal thyroid function and healthy hair growth. Low ferritin (the stored form of iron) is one of the most common causes of hair loss in women, so always ask your doctor to test both your iron and ferritin levels.

Fatigue: Since your body's energy production is dependent on normal levels of thyroid hormone, an underactive thyroid will create severe fatigue.

Poor digestive function: Poor thyroid function slows the transit of food through the intestines, resulting in gas, bloating, decreased bowel movements, and an overall sense that the food is just sitting in the gut and not moving through properly.

Problems with male fertility: Hypothyroidism in men decreases sex drive and causes impotence and low sperm count.

Miscarriage: When thyroid function is low, it is common for progesterone levels to be low, resulting in an increased tendency for miscarriage.

Slow metabolism: Hypothyroidism slows the body's overall metabolism and fat-burning processes, making it harder for the body to burn fat by shutting down the sites on the cells that respond to lipase, an enzyme that metabolizes fat.

Stunted growth in children: The incidence of hypothyroidism is now increasing in children at a rate similar to that of adults. A low thyroid can interfere with normal growth and development and even put puberty on hold. The risk is four times higher in girls than in boys.

Poor glucose metabolism: Glucose metabolism is the rate at which the body uses glucose to make energy. The brain is the most important consumer of glucose, so when glucose metabolism is poor, you get brain fog. People with low thyroid function absorb glucose more slowly than normal, and their cells don't use it to make energy as readily. This creates problems with blood sugar, such as hypoglycemia, and produces symptoms of fatigue, irritability, and light-headedness. The problem is not that there is too little glucose in the blood, but rather that the glucose can't get into the cells.

High blood sugar: Hyperthyroidism, creating excessive thyroid hormones, causes increased glucose production in the liver; rapid absorption of glucose from the intestines, raising the blood sugar; and increased insulin resistance where the body cannot utilize insulin efficiently.

High cholesterol and triglyceride levels: Hypothyroidism makes the liver and gallbladder sluggish, so fat is not easily metabolized and cleared from the body, allowing cholesterol and triglycerides to accumulate in the blood. In fact, in his groundbreaking 1976 book *Hypothyroidism: The Unsuspected Illness,* Dr. Broda O. Barnes presented research showing that the cardiovascular complications of diabetes are due to low thyroid function rather than insulin.

Problems with high estrogen/low progesterone: Low thyroid function leads to sluggish liver detoxification and delayed emptying of the gallbladder, preventing the removal of estrogen from the body. Moreover, when the thyroid is sluggish the patient cannot make enough progesterone or the progesterone cannot gain entrance into cells. And finally, in cases of prolonged stress (a common cause of thyroid problems), the high cortisol levels prevent the formation of progesterone. This creates a situation of high estrogen/low progesterone, which can cause fibroids, cystic breasts, breast cancer, ovarian cysts, thyroid nodules, midcycle bleeding, heavy menstrual bleeding, or long menstrual cycles.

Acid reflux: Bile neutralizes stomach acids as they come into the duodenum. When bile is too thick to flow or is delayed, the digestive juices traveling through the intestines remain acidic, burning both the friendly bacteria and the lining of the gut. At the same time, the lower esophageal sphincter loosens and motility in the lower part of the esophagus slows when the thyroid gland is underactive, allowing the acidic contents of the stomach to percolate up into the esophagus, causing acid reflux.

Swelling in the legs, ankles, and feet: Low thyroid function can create swelling or edema in these areas since kidney function is depressed when the thyroid is sluggish.

Insomnia, anxiety, heartbeat arrhythmias, depression, memory loss, coldness in the body, poor circulation, inability to concentrate: These are the many symptoms of a vata disturbance, which ultimately is a signal of disrupted thyroid function.

Restless legs syndrome (RLS): The latest research shows that a combination of low iron levels and high thyroid hormone levels (as seen in hyperthyroidism or pregnancy) combine to decrease the amount of dopamine formation in the brain, contributing to RLS.

ADRENAL GLAND WEAKNESS

The adrenal glands are responsible for our "fight or flight" response to stress. When stress is prolonged and the adrenals are forced to work overtime, they can become exhausted, leading to what is commonly called adrenal fatigue or adrenal weakness.

Hans Selye, a Canadian endocrinologist, was the first to identify the three stages of adrenal gland exhaustion. He described the different stages of stress we may go through, known as the general adaptation syndrome (GAS), and how the body responds in each of these three stages. Experimenting with lab rats at McGill University in Montreal, he was able to observe a series of physiological changes in the rats after they were exposed to stressful events. After much experimentation, Selye identified these changes as a typical response anyone might have to stress and described the stages as alarm, resistance, and exhaustion.

He went on to measure one's tolerance to stress when faced with a difficult situation, calling it one's "resistance to stress," which depicts one's ability to be relaxed and composed when faced with repeated difficult situations without becoming hopeless or helpless.

Stage 1: Alarm, which is an initial drop in resistance to stress. The alarm reaction stage refers to the initial symptoms the body experiences when under stress, causing your heart rate to increase and your adrenal glands to release cortisol, giving you a boost of adrenaline and energy to run from the danger.

Stage 2: Resistance, where there is an average resistance to stress. In this stage, after the initial shock of a stressful event and having a fight-or-flight response, the body begins to repair itself, releasing less amounts of cortisol, allowing your heart rate and blood pressure to go back down to normal. During this recovery stage the body is still on high alert just in case another stress comes your way. If the stressors are resolved, then the body continues to repair itself until your hormone levels, heart rate, and blood pressure go back to the prestress state.

However, if the stressful situations continue unabated and your body remains on high alert, it has to adapt and now learn how to live with this constant high stress level. This can cause your body to go through changes to attempt to cope with the unending stress pattern, and you continue to release the stress hormone cortisol, causing your blood pressure to remain elevated. During this stage you will feel irritability, frustration, and poor concentration. If this period continues for too long without any decreases in the severity of the stress, it can lead to the exhaustion stage.

Most of the patients I see with adrenal gland exhaustion describe several months, if not years, of "burning the candle at both ends" or describe themselves as "high energy." They barrel through the days long into the wee hours of the night, accomplishing task after task with unbounded energy, not realizing that they are abusing their adrenal glands and setting the stage for the burnout that invariably follows.

Stage 3: Exhaustion, where resistance to stress is lost. This final stage is the result of prolonged and chronic stress, draining your physical, emotional, and mental resources to the point where your body no longer has the resources to combat stress. You may feel hopeless, like you want to give up, as you no longer have any strength to fight the battle. This is the stage where you will feel fatigue, burnout, depression, anxiety, and an overall decreased tolerance to stress.

Selye's book, *The Stress of Life,* first published in 1956, laid the foundation for mind-body medicine. He was a three-time Nobel Prize nominee for his work documenting the role of stress hormones on the body.

The list of symptoms that result from exhausted adrenals is almost identical to those for hypothyroidism:

- Exhaustion
- Slowed metabolism
- Feeling cold often
- Decreased immunity
- Brain fog
- Depression/anxiety
- Infertility
- PMS
- Belly fat accumulation

- Low blood pressure, dizziness when standing, low blood sugar in between meals
- Hypoglycemia
- Salt cravings
- Feeling overwhelmed or unable to cope with stress
- Sensitivity to light

The majority of the patients I see suffer from adrenal gland exhaustion, yet modern medicine has no treatment for it. There are some integrative doctors who put their patients on low levels of cortisone for a year or more to help the adrenal glands "kick back in." This approach is catastrophic. I've seen scores of people struggling to regain their adrenal gland function as they try to wean off the cortisone. I offer a serious warning: this approach only makes matters worse. Many of the patients I've seen who completed this therapy were hospitalized and could not regain their adrenal function because their adrenal glands had shut down; with the prescribed hormones flooding the body, there was no need for their adrenals to function. Trying to reawaken the glands after a year or more on these hormones is nearly impossible. The best way to regenerate the adrenal glands is to obtain proper rest. We do have some specific herbs, dietary routines, and other techniques to support the adrenal glands, but rest is the primary treatment. And as a precautionary note: when you are involved in the unending throes of stress, try to rest as much as you can during this time to prevent yourself from going through the three stages until your adrenal glands are totally exhausted and you are confined to bedrest. Following the guidelines as described below will help you get through prolonged stress, avoiding the burnout that might otherwise occur.

REST AND RECUPERATION FOR THE ADRENALS AND THYROID

The ancient doctors of Ayurveda recommended proper diet and proper bedtime as the foundations for perfect health, and they noted that, in fact, most imbalances in the physiology begin with improper diet and late bedtime. They recommended going to bed no later than 10 p.m. The adrenal glands, in particular, need rest in the hours before midnight in order to heal. Thus, you could get eight hours of sleep, going to bed at 2 a.m. and waking up at 10 a.m., and still feel exhausted.

Even if you are tired, we recommend avoiding stimulants such as caffeine. They only push the adrenal glands more, weakening them in the long run. The same holds true for white table sugar.

To support both the thyroid and the adrenals, follow a vata-pacifying diet as described in chapter 3, consisting of warm, cooked foods that incorporate good-quality fruits and vegetables, dairy products, fats, and proteins.

Use ghee (clarified butter) in your cooking to provide the cholesterol your adrenal glands need to make their hormones. If you are not lactose intolerant, drink warm milk to calm vata, allowing the endocrine system to heal. In fact, I think hot boiled milk is perhaps the most calming food you can consume, because tryptophan is produced when you boil milk. Tryptophan forms serotonin, a neurotransmitter that controls anxiety, happiness, and mood. Serotonin also produces a deep and restful sleep.

AYURVEDIC HERBS TO BALANCE THE ADRENAL AND THYROID GLANDS

The Ayurvedic herbs listed below all help to balance the adrenal and thyroid glands, contributing to the overall health and well-being of the body and mind. The herbs at the beginning of this list are those most commonly used and most broadly effective, with lesser known and used herbs coming toward the end. However, all of these herbs should be familiar to any Ayurvedic practitioner and fairly accessible to everyone.

Ashwagandha (Withania somnifera)

In Sanskrit, the name *ashwagandha* means "the smell of a horse," in reference to the fact that the herb imparts the vigor and strength of a stallion. It is frequently referred to as "Indian ginseng" because of its rejuvenating effects on the endocrine system (thyroid, adrenals, reproductive glands). It is famous for balancing thyroid hormones.

Hundreds of studies have shown the healing benefits of this herb. It boosts the immune system, helps combat the effects of stress, improves learning and memory, improves reaction time, reduces anxiety and depression without causing drowsiness, helps reduce the degeneration of brain cells, stabilizes blood sugar, lowers cholesterol, enhances sexual potency for both men and women, improves the quality of sperm, and possesses anti-inflammatory and antimalarial qualities.

Because it can contribute to deeper sleep, ashwagandha can rejuvenate the entire endocrine system. Remember, the glandular system has a very difficult time recharging when the nervous system is wound up. Thus a good night's sleep is imperative for proper endocrine functioning.

Ashwagandha also calms the nervous and endocrine system, pacifying our stress response. As we have already discussed, the adrenal glands release cortisol when we are under stress, and chronically high cortisol levels contribute to immune system weakness, high blood pressure, high blood sugar, and other physiological problems. As previously mentioned, most people are existing in a state of chronic stress, constantly calling on their adrenal glands to release more cortisol to get them through their busy days, ultimately culminating in severe fatigue as the adrenal glands become exhausted. Ashwagandha can both prevent and heal this severe level of chronic fatigue, not by pushing the glandular system to create more energy, but because it can actually prevent the fight-or-flight response by promoting feelings of calm even amidst stress. Because of this property, it is widely used for both hyper- and hypothyroidism (and hyper- and hypoadrenia).

Ashwagandha is considered the primary adaptogenic herb used in Ayurveda to protect the glandular system from the effects of prolonged stress.

Tulsi (Ocimum sanctum)

Next to ashwagandha, tulsi is perhaps the second most frequently prescribed adaptogenic herb. It is considered one of the most sacred plants in India and is known as "the queen of the herbs" due to its restorative and spiritual properties. Virtually every family home in India grows tulsi in an earthenware pot. In ancient times as tulsi traveled westward toward Europe it became known to Christians as "sacred" or "holy" basil and became included in offerings and worship rituals, looked upon as a gift of Christ.

Holy basil helps your body adapt to stressors of any kind, such as chemical, physical, infectious, and emotional. It increases endurance and has been shown in human and animal studies to reduce stress, sexual problems, sleep problems, forgetfulness, and exhaustion. People who take holy basil report less anxiety, stress, and depression. It is used for adrenal fatigue, hypothyroidism, unbalanced blood sugar, and anxiety.

Because it is antibacterial, antiviral, antifungal, and anti-inflammatory it is also used to prevent infections such as bronchitis and pneumonia.

Overall, it is one of the best remedies to enhance the body's ability to maintain balance in a stressful world.

Shilajit

Shilajit, also known as mineral pitch, known in India as the "destroyer of weakness." Dr. John Douillard, Ayurvedic author and practitioner, best describes how shilajit came to be and why it holds special life-giving properties:

About 50 million years ago, the Indian continent collided into Asia and formed the Himalayan mountain range. As the mountains formed, tropical forests were crushed and compacted between massive boulders.

The compressed forests gradually transformed into a nutrient- and mineral-rich biomass loaded with powerful humic and fulvic acids.

Now, every summer as the mountains warm, India's most prized herbal remedy literally oozes from these biomass resins in the high mountain crevasses.

Known as shilajit, this resinous and nutrient-rich biomass has been touted for millennia by Ayurveda's *Materia Medica* as the best carrier of energy and nutrition into the human body. Modern science has recently proven this by identifying fulvic and humic acids, which are found in abundance in shilajit, as the main substances responsible for energy production within the cell.

For example, shilajit can stop the abnormal buildup of tau proteins that triggers brain cell damage, supporting memory and preventing Alzheimer's.

Researchers have determined that shilajit acts at the cellular level to improve ATP production at its source, inside the mitochondria. The ATP molecule is the unit of currency for cellular energy; it is the means by which cells store and transport energy. If the mitochondria are malfunctioning, your cells cannot produce enough energy, making it difficult for your body to perform its normal tasks. Shilajit has been shown to prevent mitochondrial dysfunction, allowing you to experience abundant energy throughout the day. In one recent study, after undergoing tremendous amounts of exercise, mice that were not given shilajit depleted their energy twice as fast compared to the group that were given it.

Shilajit is also known to enhance fertility because it has profound effects on the hormonal system. In one study, men receiving shilajit twice a day demonstrated significantly higher testosterone levels compared to a placebo group. It is widely known that shilajit can boost the body's production of hormones that typically decline with age, allowing the body to respond as it once did when it was younger.

Since they are basically formed from dirt, fulvic and humic acids contain many nutrients that improve gut health, boosting the ability of the friendly bacteria to repopulate and form a healthy microbiome environment. Soil-based probiotics have only recently become an important part of the arsenal of both holistic and allopathic doctors. Soil-based microorganisms have an outer shell that is naturally resistant to the acids in the stomach and upper digestive tract. When these probiotics are ingested, they travel all the way to the lower intestine. Thus, shilajit, a source of nutrients for these soil-based microorganisms, is known to encourage the growth of probiotics throughout the entire gut.

Shilajit is known as a *yoga vahi,* which means that it can drag other nutrients into cells, enhancing their absorption. This is because the fulvic acid molecule is so small that it is able to penetrate cells and reach the mitochondria. In fact, fulvic acid is known as a "nutrient booster" because it can help us absorb and use many nutrients, such as probiotics, antioxidants, electrolytes, fatty acids, and minerals. One study showed that coenzyme Q10 (which boosts energy in the heart, liver, and kidneys) gained 29 percent better delivery into cells when combined with shilajit, thus enhancing stamina and performance and protecting the heart against free radicals. This is why ashwagandha, one of the best herbs to support both the thyroid gland and the adrenal glands, is commonly used in combination with shilajit to create a powerful formulation for a weak thyroid.

Kanchanar (Bauhinia variegata)

Kanchanar is widely used in Ayurveda not only for balancing the thyroid gland but also for any glandular enlargements, such as uterine fibroids, cysts (including polycystic ovaries), lipomas, tumors, cancer, and goiters. It is even used for swelling of the prostate gland in men, and it is great for healing wounds, fistulas, and boils. It is the most common herb used to reduce swelling in the neck and goiter. It helps flush the lymphatic system of toxins, sluggishness, and accumulated wastes, with specific benefits for the thyroid gland, and is especially useful for the treatment of obesity associated with hypothyroidism. It also maintains balance in thyroid hormone production by increasing levels if they become too low or decreasing levels if they become too high. For this reason, it is used for both hypo- and hyperthyroidism.

We have patients take kanchanar internally or externally—in the latter case they rub a transdermal kanchanar cream directly on their thyroid gland to shrink swelling of the gland or nodules.

Patrang (Caesalpinia sappan)

Patrang is an extremely versatile herb that can be used to rebalance the adrenals, thyroid, or ovaries. It is indicated for both hyperactivity (when the glands are releasing too many hormones due to high levels of stress) and hypoactivity (when the glands are now exhausted and can't release enough of their hormones) of any of these glands and can be used at any age, even in young children. It is used to both bring on the menstrual cycle and regulate the cycle after childbirth and has the unique qualities of balancing both a heavy and a scanty menstrual flow. It also supports liver function and protects the liver from damage, which, as we've discussed, is vital to balancing thyroid function.

Coleus (Coleus forskohlii)

Coleus forskohlii, commonly known as *forskolin* (sometimes called *pashan bhed*), stimulates the production of T4 and T3 thyroid hormones and at the same time enhances the proper uptake of iodine into the thyroid cells.

It also stimulates the production of a molecule called cyclic AMP (cAMP). In our bodies, cyclic AMP helps our cells talk to each other. One example of this is that cAMP is needed for the transmission of information in the hypothalamic-pituitary axis aiding in the production of TSH. It also instructs the cells to increase the production of hormone-sensitive lipase, an enzyme that burns fat. Thus by both stimulating the release of thyroid hormone and increasing the basal metabolism, allowing more calories to be burned at rest, this herb is famous for counteracting hypothyroidism and helping the body burn fat and calories.

5

Hashimoto's Thyroiditis

Autoimmune Disease of the Thyroid Gland

Melanie came to see me a couple of years ago. This once vibrant woman had become a housebound invalid at the age of thirty-five. A few minutes in the sun left her with a weeping rash all over her body. A simple walk down a grocery-store aisle stocked with laundry detergents brought on debilitating nausea. Virtually every food made her retch.

In the months before her visit, Melanie's endocrinologist had diagnosed her with Hashimoto's disease, an autoimmune condition in which the thyroid gland undergoes relentless attacks from the body's own misfiring immune system, destroying it over time. Blood work showed her thyroid antibody levels were through the roof. Her doctor prescribed Synthroid, a synthetic version of thyroid hormone. Understandably anxious, Melanie asked her endocrinologist when she should get retested to see if her antibody levels would decrease with her new treatment, to which the doctor responded, "Don't bother, because the levels will never come down for the rest of your life. It's not even worth checking."

In a sense, the doctor was right. Melanie's thyroid would not improve with just the administration of hormones. Melanie, like all patients with Hashimoto's, needed a comprehensive treatment plan, one that addressed her body as a whole, that evaluated all the influences on her health, from diet and bedtime to daily stressors, and that went to the core of her problem: her faulty immune system. Only then, with the appropriate use of herbs, dietary changes, and detoxification, could Melanie get (and stay) better.

Over the course of the next year Melanie dove into her new Ayurvedic treatment protocol, eagerly looking for any signs of relief from her debilitating symptoms. She diligently followed her regime and learned how to recalibrate the three parts of her immune system, which entailed regrowing her friendly gut bacteria, which had been ravaged in her youth by frequent rounds of antibiotics; carefully cleaning her liver from the insults of past consumption of fast foods; and removing festering toxins from her bone marrow (using the herbs and foods described in this chapter), which were wreaking havoc on her immune system.

The first thing Melanie noticed as the months went by was that she was able to eat some of the foods that had previously bothered her. As time went on, she was able to slowly add back more and more of the previously offending foods, much to her delight. Next, she realized that sunlight no longer bothered her skin, and she felt ecstatic when she was able to play volleyball on the beach with her friends for the first time in a long while. She was shocked when she was able to go to the supermarket and tolerate even the strongest chemical scents in the cleaning product aisles.

Perhaps the best part of all was that after one year of treatment, her thyroid antibodies dropped more than 100 points, and then they dropped another 150 points in the second year, bringing her levels to within a few points of the normal range! Now she knew she was on the mend, and finally on the path back to vibrant health, after having been an invalid for several years.

Melanie is far from alone. In the United States, autoimmune disease strikes one in five people, 75 percent of whom are women. Starker yet, autoimmune disease accounts for 90 percent of hypothyroidism, mostly due to Hashimoto's thyroiditis, named after a Japanese physician from before World War I.

As is evident from Melanie's case, Hashimoto's takes a toll. It starts with swelling in the throat and can cause a range of unpleasant effects, such as puffiness in the face, fatigue, weight gain, memory loss, constipation, depression, enlarged tongue, dry skin—and that's only the beginning. Melanie's case is a depiction of typical Hashimoto's patients. First their blood work shows high levels of thyroid antibodies. Next they are immediately prescribed thyroid hormone. Thereafter, routine blood work is ordered periodically to check hormone levels and make adjustments to the dosage of medicine. And when they are still not feeling well, more medications are given for each symptom they describe: depression, arrhythmias, acid reflux, hair loss, weight gain, and osteoporosis.

This chapter will describe effective tools in the treatment of Hashimoto's disease, so that you can shift your focus from treatment of the thyroid to fixing the misguided immune system—which necessarily involves paying attention to sleep habits and bedtime, digestion/gut health, elimination, diet, toxin exposure, and stress levels. These and other issues have been examined throughout the book. If you ignore these factors, your results will be minimal at best.

The therapies outlined in this chapter need to be implemented as soon as possible to prevent irreversible damage to the thyroid gland, which would necessitate the use of thyroid hormone. Early detection and treatment of the various parts of the immune system are important to get their functions back on track. As the immune system slowly starts to regain its intelligence and its attacks on the thyroid gland decrease, support is then given to the thyroid gland so it can once again make adequate levels of hormones, usually negating the need for supplemental thyroid hormone.

WHAT IS THE IMMUNE SYSTEM?

Human beings coexist with millions of bacteria, viruses, and other microbes. Some of these microbes are beneficial to us or to our environment. Others, should they enter our bodies or proliferate beyond normal levels, can cause us harm. The immune system is our protective force; normally it protects us from these pathogens by keeping them out or at least under control.

The immune system is divided into two parts. The first part comprises the defenses you are born with, known as the *innate* system. The second part, the *adaptive* or *acquired* immune system, develops as you grow and come into contact with pathogenic organisms. Once your immune system has encountered a particular pathogen, it will remember it, and if you should encounter that pathogen again, your immune system will recognize it the second time around, allowing your body to respond more quickly to fight off infection. Measles is a good example; once you contract and conquer this common childhood illness, you gain lifelong immunity to it.

The innate part of the immune system comes into play immediately upon the appearance of an antigen in or on the body. An antigen is any substance that causes your immune system to produce antibodies—it may be a chemical from the environment, bacteria, viruses, or pollen, for example. Your skin, for instance, is part of the innate immune system, providing a waterproof barrier that prevents pathogens from entering your body. The mucous membranes in your nose and mouth produce sticky mucus that can trap bacteria and other pathogens. The highly acidic gastric juices produced by your stomach help kill off many of the bacteria that enter our systems from the food we eat. Even the saliva in your mouth can reduce the amount of bacteria and other pathogens found there.

If bacteria or other pathogens manage to get through these first-line defenses, they will encounter a second line of defense present in your blood (via specialized white blood cells) or in chemicals released by your cells and tissues. The white blood cells—such as neutrophils, lymphocytes, eosinophils, monocytes, and basophils—encounter pathogens in the blood. Neutrophils engulf and destroy bacteria with special chemicals. Eosinophils and monocytes swallow foreign particles, and basophils create inflammation.

Inflammation that occurs when your body is fighting infections and pathogens is normal. Tissues damaged by bacteria, trauma, toxins, or heat release chemicals such as histamine and prostaglandins that cause blood vessels to leak fluid into the tissues, causing swelling. The inflammation that occurs as the body is fighting infection is fine for the occasional acute, short-lived assaults. But problems set in when an infection becomes chronic (such as with yeast infections or SIBO in your gut), combined with an unhealthy diet, exposure to pesticides, heavy metals, and other toxins, or too much stress. Then our immune systems can enter a hyperreactive state, the foundation for all autoimmune diseases.

This chapter will focus primarily on three specific parts of the immune system that play a vital role in normal immune function: the gut flora, the liver, and the bone marrow. When the immune system works well, we are well. When it doesn't, no amount of thyroid hormone will repair the gland and restore health.

THE THREE PARTS OF THE IMMUNE SYSTEM

The Friendly Gut Bacteria

When babies are born, their gut is sterile and "leaky," with little perforations in the intestinal lining. As mothers begin breastfeeding their babies, friendly bacteria begin to grow in their gut. A crucial substance is released during the first two days of breastfeeding: colostrum, which "seals" these little holes in the gut, so that when the milk comes through on the third day, it won't "leak" through, which could cause the immune system to mount an attack, causing food allergies and sensitivities.

It is extremely important that nothing interferes with the growth of these delicate flora during the early childhood years, so your child can develop a normal functioning immune system, one that is strong enough to protect against the invading organisms that enter the mouth and nasal passages with every breath, yet balanced enough to know not to attack food or bodily tissues.

However, with each immunization or round of antibiotics, the friendly bacteria are wiped out, and with chronic exposure to these types of pharmaceuticals, they become unable to regenerate adequately. This creates a fertile breeding ground for the growth of unwanted pathogenic organisms in the digestive tract, setting up the conditions for the overgrowth of *Candida albicans* yeast.

Why is it important to keep yeast in check? Our intestines happily host small amounts of yeast. But if their surveillance team, the gut flora, are destroyed, the yeast is left unchecked, now multiplying as much as it wants, and eventually it migrates out of your digestive tract, spreading throughout the body. As it travels out of the gut, it makes little perforations, creating what is known as a "leaky gut," which now allows food to escape the intestines. Food particles anywhere other than the digestive tract are considered invaders by the immune system. Once it begins to identify these foods as invaders, you become prone to food allergies and sensitivities, chronic inflammation, and a hyperreactive immune system, creating fertile conditions for autoimmune disease.

The modern medical approach to treating yeast infections is to use medications such as nystatin and Diflucan or other antifungal medications. Some even prescribe antibiotics.

More holistically oriented practitioners often try to starve yeast overgrowth to death by following restrictive diets, avoiding any foods that could feed yeast. They may also try to kill the yeast using natural remedies like pau d'arco tea, berberine, grapefruit seed extract, caprylic acid, and garlic.

I have treated thousands of yeast infections through my years of practice, and I found early on that none of these approaches are necessary and, in fact, work either temporarily or not at all. Starving the yeast to death doesn't work because you end up starving the patient as well, since just about every food known to humankind will feed yeast. And trying to kill the yeast using either the pharmaceuticals or the natural remedies will end up killing the yeast . . . and the friendly bacteria as well, allowing the yeast to promptly regrow!

The best approach is to repopulate the gut with beneficial bacteria using a good-quality probiotic or high-quality homemade yogurt (I recommend the ProTren brand; see page 62). Once they reach sufficient numbers, these friendly bacteria in the gut will kill the yeast for you. Thus, the goal is not to kill organisms in the gut but instead to create an environment where "the bad guys leave," as Dr. Mishra always told me.

You might also try slippery elm tea. This beneficial herb heals the lining of the gut, which encourages the growth of the good bacteria, much like bringing new topsoil into your garden. This type of prebiotic is important because overuse of certain pharmaceuticals depletes not only the friendly bacteria but the lining of the gut as well, making it difficult for the friendly bacteria to grow. This is why some people have a hard time regrowing their friendly bacteria: they may have a good probiotic, but it is like planting seeds in sandy soil—they won't take.

ॐ Slippery Elm Tea

Combine ½ teaspoon of slippery elm bark with 1 quart of water. Bring to a boil, cover, and boil for 5 minutes, then turn off the heat and let steep for at least 20 minutes. Strain out the bark. Sip over the next 4 hours, drinking up to 4 cups a day. Make a fresh batch each day. Continue this regimen for at least the first 6 months of your Hashimoto's treatment protocol.

The friendly bacteria in our gut (all 100 trillion of them) form the foundation of our health. They break down and absorb nutrients from the food we eat and are the first line of defense against cold and flu viruses. The latest research shows that they even have a beneficial effect on our brain chemistry. So let's take a moment to explore, through an Ayurvedic lens, the heralded gut-brain connection.

We tend to think of the central nervous system as comprising the brain and spinal cord. But the digestive tract is home to the enteric nervous system, which contains more than 100 million nerve cells. That's more than the spinal cord! (This information comes to us through the wonders of modern science. But stop to consider that, well before the invention of microscopes, the early doctors of Ayurveda recognized the role of friendly bacteria in our brain chemistry.)

Friendly bacteria produce an astonishing 90 percent of the neurotransmitters in our brains. The implications are just as astounding. The ancient seers warned us to take heed when apana vata, home to the friendly bacteria, falls out of balance and impinges on prana vata, site of the brain. We see the real-world consequences—hyperactivity, sensory and motor delays, autistic spectrum disorders, food allergies, and alarming rates of autoimmune disease—all around us in children who take loads of antibiotics and receive up to seventy immunizations at an early stage in their development.

Clinically I see this on a daily basis. Usually patients who present with numerous food allergies, leaky gut, inflammation, and autoimmune diseases have a history of frequent use of antibiotics, birth control pills, proton pump inhibitors (antacid drugs), steroids, and nonsteroidal anti-inflammatory medications along with numerous rounds of immunizations. Over time these medications wreak havoc on the immune system as they destroy the delicate, life-giving friendly bacteria, creating the conditions chronicled above.

In our office we instruct patients to avoid foods to which they are allergic or sensitive until we can balance the good versus the bad bacteria in their gastrointestinal tracts. Generally we direct our Hashimoto's patients to avoid gluten, whose molecules resemble thyroid tissue, both of which will receive attacks by virtue of a hyperreactive immune system. Once we fix all three parts of their immune systems through dietary changes, herbal treatments, and correct detoxification, the food sensitivities recede and patients can usually go back to eating the foods that had previously bothered them.

The Liver

Let us now consider the liver, which the ancient doctors viewed as the most important organ in the body. Bespeaking its importance, the liver performs an exhaustive list of functions. In a miraculous display of versatility, this organ manufactures enzymes responsible for blood clotting, produces a quart of bile every day to aid in the digestion of fats and the absorption of fat-soluble vitamins into your bloodstream, and stores and releases glucose for energy when your blood sugar gets too low. It breaks down excess estrogen and escorts it out of the body so you don't form cystic breasts or ovaries, not to mention fibroids. It also filters and purifies your blood system. At any point in time 15 percent of your body's total blood supply is being filtered by the liver! And the liver has an amazing capacity to regenerate itself—as little as 25 percent of the original liver mass can regenerate back to its full size.

As if the liver were not busy enough, it plays a key role in immune function. Compared with other organs, it is particularly enriched with cells of the innate immune system, and this is where foreign antigens from the gastrointestinal tract first encounter attacks from the immune system. The immune system's macrophages (killer cells) start out in the bone marrow and mature in the liver once they migrate there. The name *macrophages* derives from the Greek for "big eaters"; these large cells are the first on the scene as they engulf the antigen and work in tandem with other immune system cells to surround and destroy the intruder.

As we have discussed, detoxification occurs in the liver. Pharmaceuticals, nutraceuticals, alcohol, and other chemicals all pass through the liver. When overtaxed with the work of removing these acidic toxins from our bodies, the liver becomes inflamed. And it is this overheating that causes the immune system to hyperreact and create an autoimmune response.

Studies have correlated improper liver function with thyroid disease, including autoimmune Hashimoto's. According to a 1984 study published by R. R. Babb in the *American Journal of Gastroenterology,* thyroid function tests improve as liver inflammation resolves.

It is unfortunate that patients and doctors alike don't give much thought to the liver except when diagnosable diseases like hepatitis or cirrhosis develop. The truth is that these diseases don't develop overnight. It takes a long time for the small insults to build up from frequently eating junk food, consuming alcohol and other stimulants, the application of chemical-laden skin-care products, breathing polluted air, taking prescription drugs or nutraceuticals, and so on. As a busy clinician who feels the pulses of thousands of people every year, I can categorically tell you that *every* patient I see, even small children, has some degree of liver stress. It is apparent in their pulses. Given the heavy load we place on this beleaguered organ, is it any wonder that autoimmune diseases are at epidemic levels? The point is, we have to take better care of it or risk the consequences.

Before you get too depressed, I have some good news for you: the liver is great at rejuvenating itself. In fact, the liver is the only visceral organ that possesses this remarkable ability. With most organs, such as the heart, the damaged tissue is replaced with scar tissue, just like when we sustain a wound to our skin. Once scar tissue has developed, it is very difficult to reverse. The liver, however, is able to replace damaged tissue with new cells. And it can do so in fairly quick order. It can double in size in as little as three to four weeks, regenerating itself after surgical or chemical injury. This means that you can heal and restore proper function of your liver through healthy diet and appropriate herbs, which we address in various chapters throughout the book.

The Bone Marrow

Our bone marrow is where new blood cells are produced. It contains two types of stem cells: hemopoietic (which produce blood cells) and stromal (which produce fat, cartilage, and bone). This is where our white and red blood cells and platelets are made. Lymphocytes, one particular type of white blood cell that attacks viruses and pathogens are divided into T and B cells. The T cells mature in the thymus gland, whereas the B cells mature in the bone marrow.

Toxins burrowing into the bone marrow is yet another formula for autoimmune disease. Be aware of the culprits: heavy metals (from mercury/silver amalgams, air pollution, fish, immunizations containing aluminum or mercury, and air pollution caused by coal-fired power plants), pesticides, and chemicals found in our food, such as artificial sweeteners and preservatives. There are numerous pharmaceuticals that make their way into the bone marrow as well, as described in a 2000 study in *Immunopharmacology,* "Drugs Toxic to the Bone Marrow that Target the Stromal Cells." The stromal cells are the cells in the bone marrow that support its function.

It is of utmost importance to keep our bone marrow clean and functioning properly. However, these modern environmental chemicals and pharmaceuticals easily make their way into this tissue, disrupting its function. Think of it this way: if virtually all of your immune system cells are born in the bone marrow, starting out their lives as stem cells and then maturing into platelets, white blood cells, and red blood cells, then any toxin reaching there will disturb the formation of these cells, creating cancer and autoimmune diseases.

A 2013 article in *Experimental and Toxicologic Pathology* demonstrated how inhalation of toxic pesticides causes diseases due to their accumulation in the bone marrow. In fact, numerous other studies have proven how environmental toxins make their way into the marrow, creating serious disease.

I personally have had several patients who developed intractable leukemia, went to the Mayo Clinic for evaluation, and were told it was caused by pharmaceuticals they were taking, which in their words, "scarred the bone marrow."

We have to keep in mind that most of the hundreds of environmental toxins are new on the scene, and our bodies have not developed the capacity to ward them off; thus we suffer the consequences as these potent chemicals make their way into our delicate bone marrow, disrupting its function. If you recall from our earlier discussion on the seven tissues, we can actually feel in the pulse how they are functioning. In addition to that, each of the four types of toxins has a very specific feel to it. Thus, we can feel, for example, when ama visha and gara visha have made their way deep into the bone marrow. And from experience, I can emphatically tell you this: most if not all of us are harboring these deadly toxins in our bone marrow. It's just a matter of time before they build up enough to create a cancer or an autoimmune condition. Fortunately, you are learning in the chapters of this book the importance of removing them before this happens.

HOW TO RECALIBRATE THE THREE PARTS OF THE IMMUNE SYSTEM

In order to treat Hashimoto's, you must learn how to get your immune system back on track so it can function properly and stop its relentless assaults on your thyroid gland. This section will give you insight into how you can accomplish this. Keep in mind that it can take months, if not a few years, to do this, but it will be well worth your effort. Most people whose immune system is malfunctioning develop more than one, in fact numerous, autoimmune diseases. This is due to the fact that therapies are usually geared toward suppressing the symptom of the particular disease, rather than fixing the immune system problems at their deepest levels. In fact, most of my autoimmune patients do indeed present with more than one autoimmune condition (one of my patients had seven!).

The good news here is whatever work you are doing for your Hashimoto's will help any other autoimmune disease you may have as well. Follow the guidelines presented here to get your immune system normalized, making sure you follow all the guidelines for diet and daily routine, to give your body optimum advantage in returning you to normal health.

1. Replenish the Gut Flora

As previously mentioned, we recommend a high-quality probiotic to help patients regrow their intestinal flora (see chapter 5). We also instruct patients to include in their diet *prebiotics*—foods that encourage the growth of friendly bacteria, much like adding fertilizer to the soil to encourage seeds to grow. A cooked apple in the morning is a good example. Apples contain pectin, which functions as a prebiotic in the gut. Because digestion is weak in the morning, we teach patients to peel and core an apple, quarter it, cover it with water in a small pot, add a clove or two, and then boil until soft. Cooking the apple makes it easier to digest, and cloves can ignite the weak digestive fire in the morning without creating too much pitta or heat.

Other prebiotics include artichokes, taro root, okra, tamarind, asparagus, burdock root, chicory root, ghee, and herbs like slippery elm. (See the recipe for slippery elm tea on page 99.)

2. Cool Down the Heat in the Liver

The liver is considered the seat of digestion, burning up and transforming food as it enters the body. As we noted in chapter 1, the ancient texts described the liver as having five flames (in order to digest and transform the five elements: space, air, fire, water, and earth). So the liver is generally a "hot" organ. When it also becomes overburdened with toxins, agni, or heat, builds up. Now any disturbance, whether another load of sugary foods, a dose of pharmaceuticals, or even just a skipped meal, sends that agni raging out of control, spilling intense heat into the entire body, creating inflammation and disturbance as it goes.

Now consider this paradox: the vast majority of herbs used to detoxify the liver heat it at the same time. Dandelion, milk thistle, and burdock root, all of which are regularly used by holistic practitioners and patients in the fad cleanses circulating on the internet, fall into this category.

Many patients have heard or read that turmeric is a strong anti-inflammatory, so they rush out to buy capsules and take them diligently every day. While turmeric does have anti-inflammatory and detoxifying capabilities, when taken in this manner it will dramatically heat the liver and upset its function, quickly backfiring on patients as they unknowingly create even more inflammation and autoimmune predisposition by stoking the liver's flames. It is best to cook with turmeric instead; see page 113.

Additionally, many practitioners put their patients on numerous remedies, failing to understand that everything we swallow has to go through the liver to be scanned. Every remedy has the overall effect of creating more heat, so the total amount of remedies a patient takes must be carefully monitored. We often find that our new patients are taking an extremely long list of pharmaceuticals, nutraceuticals, and herbs. We slowly wean them off their pharmaceuticals when we can, take them immediately off most of their nutraceuticals, and give as many of the herbs as we can transdermally (through the skin, thus bypassing the liver). We also recommend and use homeopathic dilutions of herbs (sipped slowly in water all day) and very dilute teas. We are careful to limit the amount of herbs taken orally.

To cool the liver, we recommend the following:

Clay packs: Place clay on the skin over the liver (below the ribs on the right) for 10 minutes each day to draw out the heat. You can order these from www.chandika.com.

Liver-cooling herbs: We generally recommend two Indian herbs, bhumi amla and mankand; see the profiles below.

Cooling vegetables: Food can have a medicinal effect in reducing the liver's temperature. The best vegetable for cooling heat in the liver, loki squash, is available at Indian markets. If you cannot find loki squash, good alternatives are yellow squash and green zucchini. All of them must be cooked in order to be effective at pulling heat from the liver.

ॐ Loki Squash

1 teaspoon ghee

1/4 teaspoon ground coriander

1/4 teaspoon ground cumin

1/4 teaspoon ground fennel

1/4 teaspoon ground turmeric

1 loki squash, peeled and chopped into 1-inch chunks

Melt the ghee, add the spices, and cook over a low heat for 1–2 minutes, infusing the spices into the ghee. Add the squash and cook, stirring, for another minute or two. Put on a lid, and let the squash cook in its own juices for 15 to 20 minutes until soft, adding a little spring water if necessary to avoid burning. Eat warm.

We don't recommend fasting for the purposes of cleansing because it generates heat in the liver.

3. Clean the Bone Marrow

We recommend two highly specialized herbs for cleaning bone marrow: guduchi and moringa; see the profiles below. Be careful when using them, as they are extremely powerful, and you need to be able to regulate the amount of toxins coming out of the bone marrow. Toxins exit the body through various channels and into bowel movements, urine, and sweat. If the toxins exit too quickly, they can rupture these delicate microchannels, creating a detox crisis, and concomitant health problems, by roaming freely through the body. You might suffer, for example, from rashes, eczema, and other skin conditions.

Even though guduchi is *the* main herb used to clean bone marrow, the leaves of the plant can heat the liver. Therefore, in autoimmune cases we only use the stem, the alkaline part of the plant. The stem's juice is extracted and then dried into a powder. This ancient classical remedy is called *guduchi satwa,* and it is by far the most important agent for the removal of toxins from the bone marrow.

Bone Broth

Bone broth is made by the long-term cooking of joints, cartilage, and bones in water with vegetables and herbs. This is different from a stock, which is made with more meat and in one or two hours, creating a thinner broth. Bone broth is more viscous due to the collagen that seeps out of the joints and bones during the long-term cooking, making these otherwise inaccessible nutrients more bioavailable. These nutrients (gelatin, collagen, amino acids, minerals, and protein) from the bone marrow seep into the broth and can help reverse autoimmunity in two ways: by sealing the leaky gut (bone broth contains glutamine, an amino acid that heals the gut lining) and nourishing the bone marrow.

AYURVEDIC HERBS AND OTHER TREATMENTS FOR AUTOIMMUNE THYROID DISORDERS

Bhumi Amla (Phyllanthus niruri)

Bhumi amla is one of my favorite herbs. This amazing herb cools the heat in the liver, allowing it to work properly again. It is so effective in pulling heat and inflammation out of the liver that it is widely used in the treatment of all three types of hepatitis: A, B, and C. Because it provides relief to an overheated liver, it can be used for menorrhagia (heavy menstrual flow), all autoimmune diseases, cholesterol and blood sugar problems, food allergies, and inflammation, all of which are driven by an angry hot liver. It is also one of the best remedies for headaches, since overheating in the liver accounts for most of the headaches we see (the heat in the liver rises up to the head, affecting the blood vessels there).

Use of this herb for several months cools the liver and slowly settles down the immune system, which can eliminate food allergies/sensitivities and resolve long-standing autoimmune problems. Bhumi amla is a mainstay in my practice.

Mankand (Alocasia indica)

Mankand is perhaps the only liver-cleansing herb whose effects on that organ are *only* cooling and regenerating. However, it is extremely rare and hard to find.

Years ago, a relative of my teacher, Vaidya Rama Kant Mishra, became critically ill and was in the hospital in a coma with liver failure due to cirrhosis of the liver. He was put on a waiting list for a liver transplant. His family contacted Dr. Mishra to see if he could help. He told them that mankand could potentially save the patient's life, if they could find it. Miraculously, they did. Luckily, the patient came out of his coma in a few days. When he did, he took the mankand his family had found, and his liver function then improved so much that doctors took him off the waiting list for a liver transplant. Dr. Mishra and I were teaching a course on the liver in Pennsylvania soon after, and this man flew from India to attend our course. I had the opportunity to meet him and take his pulse, witnessing firsthand his incredible recovery. I have been fortunate to find a source for this lifesaving herb for use in my own practice, and indeed, I have seen it reverse problematic liver disease, especially fatty liver and cirrhosis of the liver. I have also seen it work wonders in the treatment of autoimmune disease because of its liver-cooling properties.

Guduchi (Tinospora cordifolia)

Dr. Mishra and his father, Kameswar Mishra, both masters of Ayurveda, had encyclopedic knowledge of more than seven hundred herbs. But their favorite herb was guduchi, which they referred to as *divya aushaudhi* (divine plant) and considered the best *rasayana* (rejuvenating) herb—and the best herb for autoimmune disturbance. It is among the most highly revered herbs of Ayurvedic medicine and is categorized as one of the three *amrit,* or ambrosia plants, an indication of its elevated status as a sacred herb.

The sixteenth-century Ayurvedic treatise Bhava Prakasha, by Bhava Mishra, provides insight into the spiritual nature of guduchi by naming it *chinnodbhava,* "able to grow even when cut." Vaidya Mishra, a descendant of Bhava Mishra, elaborated further, teaching his students that guduchi possesses *amrit siddhi,* meaning that it is so full of life energy that it has the ability to grow without soil or water. He always compared it to the great yogis, who could live without food or water and instead subsisted on the pranic energy in the air.

Guduchi is widely used in Ayurveda for its detoxifying, rejuvenating, and immune-enhancing capabilities. It is now being studied and used in modern medicine for cold and flu prevention, skin disorders, allergies, inflammation, arthritis, psoriasis, eczema, high cholesterol, hepatitis, liver disorders, and gout and most recently to mitigate the effects of chemotherapy.

As we have discussed, the accumulation of toxins in bone marrow can be a trigger for both autoimmune diseases and cancer. Guduchi is one of the very few herbs that can go deeply into the bone marrow to cleanse it of toxins, and for this reason it is the absolute best herb for both preventing and treating these diseases. It is also especially useful in the treatment of all types of leukemia and other bone marrow diseases.

Moringa (Moringa oleifera)

It is believed that the moringa tree originated in northern India and was being used in Ayurvedic medicine more than five thousand years ago. There are also accounts of its being utilized by the ancient Greeks, Romans, and Egyptians. This tree was, and still is, considered a panacea, and it is referred to as the "wonder tree," the "divine tree," and the "miracle tree," among other names.

Various parts of the tree are used for medicine, especially the long pods and leaves. Considered a superfood, it boasts numerous health benefits, including antitumor, antipyretic, antiepileptic, anti-inflammatory, anti-ulcer, antispasmodic, antihypertensive, antidiabetic, antioxidant, diuretic, cholesterol-lowering, hepatoprotective, antibacterial, and antifungal activities. Whew!

As a result of its multiplicity of uses, a great deal of research is under way on moringa's phytochemical composition and pharmacological properties. It is said to contain twenty-five times more iron than spinach, seventeen times more calcium than milk, fifteen times more potassium than bananas, ten times more vitamin A than carrots, and four times more protein than milk. In addition, the leaves of the tree are loaded with antioxidants and contain quercetin, which is a natural antihistamine.

Moringa is the only other remedy besides guduchi capable of eliminating toxins from the bone marrow, which makes it an invaluable tool in both the prevention and treatment of autoimmune diseases and cancer.

There are now dozens of supplement companies selling dried and powdered moringa online. You can take it in capsule form, make a tea, or stir the dried leaves into your soups, stews, and dahls. If you can locate a good Indian grocery store, you may be able to find the fresh leaves or pods and use them in your cooking. Try "drumstick" soup (the drumstick is the pod from the moringa tree), which is tasty, nourishing, and a great remedy for any autoimmune condition; see the recipe below. There are also numerous recipes online.

ॐ Drumstick Soup

Stage One Ingredients

3 cups water

4 moringa sticks/pods, chopped into 2-inch pieces
   (fresh is best, but frozen is fine)

1 teaspoon ghee

1 teaspoon salt

¹/₄ teaspoon ground coriander

¹/₄ teaspoon ground cumin

¹/₄ teaspoon ground fennel

¹/₄ teaspoon ground turmeric

Combine all the ingredients in a pot, bring to a boil, then reduce the heat and let simmer for 30 to 40 minutes, stirring occasionally. Transfer the soup to a blender, or use a handheld immersion blender directly in the pot, and pulse 5 to 10 times. The goal is to crush the moringa sticks, not puree them.

Set a strainer over a large pot. Pour the soup through the strainer, catching the broth in the pot. Press the solids in the strainer with a spoon to extract as much of the broth as possible.

Stage Two Ingredients

1 tablespoon ghee

¹/₄ teaspoon ground cumin

¹/₄ teaspoon garam masala

6 fresh curry leaves (available from Indian markets)

2 tablespoons mung dal flour (ground-up split mung beans)

Freshly squeezed lime juice, for garnish

Chopped fresh cilantro, for garnish

Warm the ghee in a small pan over medium-high heat. Add the cumin and garam masala, and sauté until aromatic, about 1 minute. Add to the broth in the pot, along with the curry leaves.

Mix the mung dal flour with a bit of room-temperature water to make a thin, smooth paste. Stir into the broth.

Return the pot with the broth to the stovetop. Simmer for approximately 5 minutes to thicken the soup and meld the flavors. If the soup seems too thick, thin with boiling water. Serve hot, garnished with freshly squeezed lime juice and chopped cilantro.

I recommend limiting your intake of this soup to two times a week, since it is extremely effective in removing toxins.

Drumstick Soup recipe courtesy of *Ayurvedic Recipes for Balance & Bliss,* by Vaidya R.K. Mishra and Rick Talcott (Adishakti LLC, 2016)

ASHWAGANDHA AND TURMERIC: CORRECT USE FOR AUTOIMMUNE DISEASES

Both ashwagandha and turmeric have great benefit for the endocrine system and the liver, and given that fact, you might think that they would be wonderful remedies for diseases like Hashimoto's thyroiditis. However, if used incorrectly, these herbs will actually exacerbate autoimmune diseases, further heating the liver and imbalancing the thyroid. Though they can be useful in these cases, caution must be exercised.

Ashwagandha

Ashwagandha has gained great recognition in recent years, especially for its treatment of thyroid problems. Even endocrinologists are starting to recommend its use to their patients. However, it is extremely heating to the liver and will inadvertently backfire on Hashimoto's patients, as the heat it creates pushes them further into an autoimmune crisis. Therefore, though this herb can be very important for supporting the thyroid, it must be taken transdermally, in a homeopathic version diluted in a liter of water, or as a very weak tea (a pinch of herb per liter of boiled water, steeped for 20 minutes and then slowly sipped so that it comes into the liver without heating it up). See page 87 for more information about ashwagandha.

Turmeric

Turmeric has been long used in Indian and Chinese medicine for its demonstrated anti-inflammatory, antioxidant, and anticancer properties. Hundreds of research studies extol its health benefits: it kills bacteria, aids in the treatment of all cancers, prevents and slows the progression of Alzheimer's, benefits people with depression and multiple sclerosis, mitigates the symptoms of osteoarthritis and rheumatoid arthritis, and boosts the effects of chemotherapy while decreasing its side effects. Ongoing research indicates potential benefits in the treatment of pancreatic cancer and multiple myeloma. In particular, it halts the growth of blood vessels that feed cancerous tumors and heals damaged skin, making it particularly useful for psoriasis and other inflammatory skin conditions.

According to Ayurvedic texts, turmeric has hot and dry properties.

While it can be very beneficial to the liver, helping it to detoxify the blood, taking too much at once in capsule form can distress the liver. Even worse is taking the active ingredient, curcumin, on its own, which magnifies turmeric's heating side effects. Both of these remedies taken orally will aggravate autoimmune Hashimoto's.

One way to avoid the overheating quality of turmeric is to incorporate it into a spice mixture (called a *masala*) with spices that counteract its heat (see the recipe below). Another option is to cook the turmeric (or your masala) with water, ghee, dahl (lentils), and/or vegetables. The fat molecules will deliver turmeric to the fat-soluble areas of your body, and the water will deliver the turmeric to the water-soluble areas of your body. You can also simmer a pinch or two of turmeric in milk for a few minutes, which both cools its inherent heat and allows for distribution into the cells.

ॐ Masala Mix

Combine 6 parts ground coriander, 6 parts ground fennel, 1 part ground cumin, and 1 part ground turmeric. Mix well, and store in an airtight container. Use this spice mixture when you are cooking vegetables, grains, soups, chicken, dahls, and other recipes. Use ½ to 1 teaspoon, depending on how much food you are cooking.

....

Turmeric Tips

For glowing, blemish-free skin, bring 1 cup of milk to a boil, add a pinch of ground turmeric, and boil for 2 minutes. Turn off the heat, let cool, and sip slowly.

When you are sick with a cold or flu, melt 1 tablespoon of ghee in a pan over low heat. Add 1 teaspoon of turmeric, and cook, stirring constantly, for 1 minute. Pour this mixture onto your food at lunch and dinner to fight the infection. (Turmeric kills viral and bacterial infections as soon as it comes into contact with them.)

....

One final note: Turmeric is a member of the Zingiberaceae or ginger family. However, unlike ginger, the tuber or fresh root of turmeric should not be eaten raw. It is best to dry it and pulverize it into a powder. Always purchase organic turmeric.

ANTIOXIDANTS: CELLULAR PROTECTORS

Now that you have learned that environmental toxins are one of the many culprits in creating a hyperactive immune system or autoimmune disease, you must be very careful in understanding how to remove them from the body. While, yes, we need to rid our body of free radicals, we must be careful that we do so in a way that keeps the liver cool, and we must make certain that more free radicals aren't actually created in our bodies from using the artificial, man-made antioxidants commonly in use today. But first let's learn a little about free radicals and antioxidants.

When toxins enter your body from any source—pharmaceuticals, air pollution, artificial compounds found in processed foods, cigarette smoke, X-rays, pesticides, and so on—they create "oxidative stress," which means that the oxygen molecules in your body split into single atoms with unpaired electrons, called free radicals. Free radicals are highly reactive and capable of damaging cells, proteins, and even DNA. Luckily, our bodies are equipped with the equivalent of a hazmat team known as antioxidants, which halt these nasty cellular chain reactions before vital molecules are damaged.

Currently there is a "mini medical revolution" around the prevention of free radicals and oxidation. Vitamin supplement companies are manufacturing hundreds of different types of synthetic antioxidant supplements. However, clinical trials have demonstrated that synthetically produced vitamin antioxidants actually produce free radicals! This means that your daily synthetic multivitamin and mineral supplements can do more harm than good. In addition, if you take too many antioxidant supplements, you can suppress your body's own ability to turn on its own antioxidant defense system.

It is therefore best to eat as many of the antioxidant-rich foods as you can in order to help in the fight against free radicals.

Dietary Antioxidants

Many of the antioxidants at work in our body are nutrients that come from our diet. They include vitamin E (d-alpha-tocopherol), present in nuts, seeds, vegetables, fish, whole grains, and apricots; vitamin C, found in citrus fruits, green leafy vegetables, cantaloupe, kiwi, and berries; and beta-carotene, found in liver, egg yolk, milk, butter, ghee, spinach, carrots, squash, broccoli, yams, cantaloupe, peaches, and grains. Herbs and spices contain antioxidants as well.

In fact, most fruits and vegetables contain antioxidants. Ayurveda highly recommends amla berry, a prized fruit in India. It is mainly used dried, in tablet or powder form, in the United States. Amla berry, or amalaki as it is also called, has twenty times more vitamin C than an orange, yet it creates alkalinity once it is ingested, unlike synthetically derived vitamin C, which causes acidity, with side effects such as nausea, vomiting, heartburn, stomach cramps, and headaches, to name a few.

Glutathione: Mother of All Antioxidants

Glutathione is an antioxidant found in every single cell of your body. In fact, it is the only antioxidant that resides within cells. It is also known as the "mother of all antioxidants" because it recycles other antioxidants, such as vitamins C and E, once they are used up. It is even able to regenerate itself.

The highest concentrations of glutathione are in the liver, the body's main detoxification organ. The liver has two phases of detoxification: in phase one the liver converts the toxins into water-soluble compounds, making it easy to flush them out, and in phase two glutathione is used to bind those toxins so that they can be dumped into the urine or bile. If glutathione is low, toxins can build up, causing severe repercussions to your health, including autoimmune diseases and cancer.

The antioxidant and detoxifying powers in glutathione come from an amino acid, cysteine, which most Americans don't consume enough of in their diets, leading to glutathione deficiency in most people, even if they are healthy. Good dietary sources of cysteine include poultry, yogurt, egg yolks, broccoli, brussels sprouts, oats, and wheat germ. Other glutathione-rich foods include asparagus, spinach, avocado, yellow squash, green zucchini, melons, grapefruit, and peaches.

Glutathione levels also become depleted due to excessive toxins in the body; when phase two detoxification is in full swing, glutathione gets used up at a good rate. As an antioxidant, it also is put to work neutralizing free radicals in the body as needed to battle oxidative stress. So as you might imagine, in this modern era many of us have low glutathione levels.

As it turns out, glutathione is one of the major factors influencing T4 to T3 conversion, so insufficient levels would lead to thyroid problems. Because of its involvement in detoxification and liver function, it may also play a key role in autoimmune thyroid disorders. Therefore, it is of utmost importance that patients with Hashimoto's normalize their glutathione levels.

Since glutathione supplements cannot be absorbed effectively in the gastrointestinal tract, you cannot just pop a pill to get your daily requirements. It is better to apply it transdermally (through the skin), bypassing the digestive tract and delivering it directly into the bloodstream. We recommend swiping the glutathione cream down the spine, from top to bottom, twice a day for optimum results. Some practitioners recommend rubbing glutathione transdermally into the soles of the feet once a day.

Make sure that the glutathione you use is natural and not synthetic. It is hard to find but available. My favorite source of natural glutathione is through www.chandika.com (see resources section).

Bloodwork isn't an accurate assessment of glutathione levels because it oxidizes quickly outside of the body. Therefore, just try your best to keep up your intake of glutathione—most people consume only 35 mg of glutathione in the diet each day, far short of the recommended 250 mg.

The Genetic Factor

Advanced methods of DNA analysis are opening up a whole new realm in our understanding of why some of us wilt like unwatered flowers when exposed to toxins, while others seem to skate by with no apparent problem.

It turns out that more than 50 percent of the population has inherited gene mutations that can affect their abilities to detoxify, among other things. The good news is that our ancestors, who also harbored these genetic defects, survived through the ages. The bad news is that we are now immersed in a world teeming with chemicals and other toxins that our ancestors never had to fend off. So now, in this modern age, we must strive to keep our toxic load low, especially if we find out that we have these genetic insufficiencies that can hamper our detoxifying capabilities.

For example, many people lack a gene, called GSTM1 (glutathione S-transferase M1), that is crucial to making and recycling glutathione. Another gene mutation is known as MTHFR, and it looks as though there will be dozens more discovered in the not-too-distant future using DNA sampling. If you have inherited these genetic mutations, it is easy for you to wind up with a toxic overload because your glutathione stores will be used up more quickly than in people who do not have this mutation.

Knowing that you are just as likely as not to have a genetic mutation that inhibits your glutathione function, you can see why it is of utmost importance to eat as healthily as you can, to get your nutrients from food, herbs, and spices rather than supplements, and to decrease your exposure to harmful chemicals, all of which can deplete your stores of glutathione and other antioxidants.

When I talked with Dr. Mishra about the fact that DNA testing now shows that many of us have incomplete pathways of detoxification in the liver, such as those affecting the production of glutathione, he told me emphatically, "Guduchi can complete any detox pathway. Just give those patients guduchi."

As usual, he was right. Because guduchi is considered one of the most beneficial herbs in the Ayurvedic herbal repertoire, hundreds of studies have been undertaken to examine its efficacy. And sure enough, much of the research shows that guduchi can increase the production of glutathione in the liver, whether you have a genetic defect or not.

CAN LOW LEVELS OF VITAMIN D CAUSE AUTOIMMUNE DISEASES?

The vitamin D molecule was first discovered in 1920 and then classified as a vitamin, a substance essential for the normal development of the body. It wasn't until 1932 that the chemical structure of vitamin D was discovered, and at that point it was found to be a steroid hormone, known as a secosteroid, made by sunlight's action on the surface of the skin.

In recent years, there has been a dramatic decline in the vitamin D levels of Americans due to, among other factors:

- Less exposure to the sun and the increased use of sunscreens, which combine to block the formation of vitamin D
- A higher incidence of obesity, which correlates with low vitamin D levels
- Inflammatory disorders of the gastrointestinal tract, which reduce the absorption of vitamin D
- High levels of cortisol, which deplete the body's vitamin D supply

People with dark skin are more at risk for low vitamin D levels because they need longer periods of sun exposure than people with lighter skin to make the same amount of vitamin D, as the melanin pigment in their skin acts as a sunscreen.

Numerous studies have shown a correlation between low levels of vitamin D and autoimmune thyroid conditions, including Hashimoto's thyroiditis. One such study also showed that low levels of vitamin D are responsible for the growth of viruses in a variety of tissue "barrier" sites, such as the gut. Keep in mind our earlier discussions that implicated gut infections as a primary cause of inflammation in our bodies, which ultimately affects thyroid function. Other studies have found that 90 percent of people with autoimmune thyroid disease have a genetic defect that affects their ability to process vitamin D.

Much more research is needed. However, one fact is clear: low levels of vitamin D have been implicated in a range of autoimmune diseases. So it is important to get ample sun exposure, at least fifteen to twenty minutes a day in warm weather, without sunscreen. In the colder months use a transdermal form of vitamin D; this can be tolerated better than pills, which can upset the digestive tract.

SUPPORTING THE THYROID GLAND

Once you learn how to reestablish the innate intelligence of your immune system by following a protocol that promotes a healthy gut, liver, and bone marrow, you then need to support your thyroid gland, using the herbs described in chapter 4: shilajit, ashwagandha, holy basil, patrang, kanchanar, and coleus forskholii. These herbs will help heal, nourish, and nurture your thyroid back to health. To avoid having these herbs heat the liver, thereby negating the positive steps you've taken to cool the liver, take them in one of the following ways:

- **Transdermally** (through the skin): Apply a thin layer of transdermal cream down the spine twice a day.
- **As a tincture:** Combine two or three drops with a liter of spring water and sip slowly throughout the day.
- **As a dilute tea:** Boil 1 quart of water for 5 minutes, and then pour the hot water into a stainless-steel insulated thermos. Add ¼ teaspoon of the powdered herb. Seal the thermos, and let steep for 20 minutes, then sip the tea slowly over the next 4 hours.

In addition, follow the dietary guidelines described in chapter 8 to give your thyroid gland every opportunity to heal itself. In the initial stages of treatment for Hashimoto's or any other autoimmune disease, avoid gluten and dairy. Proteins in gluten and dairy are difficult to digest. Furthermore, gluten molecules resemble thyroid tissue, so if your immune system is operating in a hyperreactive state, it may end up attacking both thyroid cells and gluten molecules.

You should also eliminate any other foods you feel sensitive or allergic to until your immune system settles down. You can slowly reincorporate these foods back into your diet after several months of treatment.

If you have Hashimoto's or another autoimmune disease of the thyroid, it is best to work with a skilled Ayurvedic practitioner who has experience treating autoimmune diseases. Your Ayurvedic doctor will give you advice regarding other imbalances you may be exhibiting—remember, each person presents with a unique physiology, and therefore each patient will have a different treatment program to follow.

....

Contraindicated Methods
of Treating Autoimmune Diseases

The following are incorrect treatments for autoimmune diseases of the thyroid, such as Hashimoto's thyroiditis:

- **Milk thistle, burdock root, and dandelion root:** As stated previously, these herbs are contraindicated in the treatment of any type of autoimmune disease because they overheat the liver during cleansing, and this has the potential to backfire on patients by causing flare-ups.
- **Maple syrup/cayenne pepper cleanse:** This cleanse formula has circulated widely on the internet. We have seen victims of this cleanse repeatedly in our office. The cayenne pepper heats the blood and liver, aggravating autoimmune disease.
- **Colonics.** Aggressive flushing of the bowels can actually deplete the delicate layer of ojas in the gut and throw apana vata further out of balance, making it extremely difficult to balance hormones.

- **Onions, garlic, and asafoetida:** They too overheat the liver and aggravate autoimmune disease.
- **Alcohol and vinegar:** Again, they overheat the liver.
- **Flaxseed and flaxseed oil:** Again, they overheat the liver, and they are extremely heating to the spleen as well.
- **Large oral doses of turmeric or ashwagandha:** Both have great benefit for the liver and endocrine system respectively, but taking large doses orally (in capsules, for example, or even in strong teas) will simply heat the liver further.
- **Fasting:** It is important to rid the body of toxins that can disturb immune function, but fasting is never recommended in these cases because the liver heats up without food to digest.

6

Gallbladder Function and the Thyroid Gland

You may be wondering why a whole chapter of this book is devoted to a small pouch that holds bile. Though it's often overlooked, the gallbladder plays a critical role in our health. It is the hidden culprit in many illnesses, and yet patients and doctors mistakenly focus on treating the various symptoms created by a malfunctioning gallbladder rather than going directly to the source of the problem. So let's see what the gallbladder does and how it is affected by an imbalanced thyroid gland.

WHAT DOES THE GALLBLADDER DO?

Breakdown of Fats

The gallbladder is a small pouch that sits directly beneath the liver, storing the bile that is continuously made by the liver. Bile comprises bile acids and salts, phospholipids, cholesterol, pigments, water, and electrolytes that keep the solution alkaline (with a pH of about 7 to 8).

Before we eat, the gallbladder is full of bile and about the size of a small pear. As we eat, in response to digestive signals, the gallbladder squirts bile into the duodenum (the beginning of the small intestine). By the end of the meal, it is usually empty and as flat as a deflated balloon. It slowly refills with bile between meals, so that it is ready for the next round of food coming in.

Fat molecules are huge globules that are too large to be absorbed into our cells. They aren't much help to us until they are broken down and assimilated into our cells. The bile held by the gallbladder contains lecithin, which dissolves these large fat globules into small droplets. Pancreatic enzymes then surround these droplets and process them into particles that are small enough to pass through the intestinal wall into the bloodstream, where they are then taken to the cells and absorbed by them.

Breakdown of Fat-Soluble Vitamins

In a similar manner, bile from the gallbladder is also responsible for breaking down fat-soluble vitamins (A, D, E, and K) so that our cells can absorb them. As we have discussed, most people have low levels of vitamin D due to insufficient exposure to sunlight and liberal use of sunblock. However, in this case, what we have is an anatomical case of sunblock, where a sluggish gallbladder can lead to decreased absorption and assimilation of vitamin D.

Elimination of Fat-Soluble Toxins

There are two types of toxins in the body: water soluble and fat soluble. The water-soluble toxins are eliminated through urine and sweat. Fat-soluble toxins are broken down into water-soluble toxins by the liver and dumped into the bile. When the gallbladder is activated, it transmits these toxins, via the bile, through the large intestines, and eventually they are eliminated in bowel movements.

When this elimination system fails to work properly, serious toxins can be reabsorbed and reenter our blood circulation, eventually depositing in fat tissues and the brain (which is made of fat), where they can be stored for years, causing serious diseases and cancer. Constipation, loose bowel movements, gas, bloating, belching, nausea, and flatulence are signals that your biliary (liver and gallbladder) system is not functioning correctly, which means that you are likely storing fat-soluble toxins. In that instance, try a tea made from Indian sarsaparilla root, which is the best herb to both clean the fat tissue and help you digest your fats better. Drink this tea approximately five times a week for six months.

ॐ *Indian Sarsaparilla Root Tea*

Boil 1 quart of water for 5 minutes, and then pour the hot water into a stainless-steel insulated thermos. Add $1/2$ teaspoon of whole coriander seeds and $1/2$ teaspoon of Indian sarsaparilla root. Seal the thermos, and let steep for at least 20 minutes, then sip slowly over the next 4 hours.

To aid in the removal of toxins from the brain and nerve tissue (which can be particularly helpful in cases of Alzheimer's, multiple sclerosis, dementia, autism, and other neurogenic diseases), add $1/4$ teaspoon of guduchi powder to the sarsaparilla; guduchi (see page 158) is the best herb to clean nerve and brain tissue.

Elimination of Cholesterol

Our bile is also the major route for the elimination of cholesterol. Many steroid hormones, such as estrogen, are made of cholesterol, and they too have to be broken down in the bile and eliminated via bowel movements.

Alkalinization of Digestive Juices

Bile fluid is very alkaline, with a pH of about 8. This is necessary to temper the high acidity of the digestive juices. As those digestive juices enter the duodenum from the stomach, they mix with the alkalinizing bile that is squirting in from the gallbladder. If the bile does not flow readily and remains hostage in the gallbladder, the digestive juices pass through the rest of the intestines as a very acidic solution, burning not only our mucosal lining but the friendly bacteria that are trying to grow in the intestinal walls. Over time, this situation can lead to inflammation, ulcerations, and infections in the gut.

WHAT IS GALLBLADDER SLUDGE?

To reiterate, the purpose of bile is to break down fats: fats from the food you eat, fatty hormones (estrogen), fat-soluble environmental toxins, fat-soluble vitamins, and so on. But in situations where there is more fat going into the bile than the bile can handle, instead of the fat breaking down into small particles and flowing out of the gallbladder, it remains stuck there. The bile and fat then bind together to create a gelatinous, gluey sludge that gets thicker and stickier and eventually clogs up the gallbladder and ducts.

One way this can happen is if the bile remains in the gallbladder for too long. Decreased thyroid function prevents bile from emptying out of your gallbladder and is therefore one of the leading causes of biliary sludge.

Sludge can also form if you eat and drink ice-cold foods and beverages (ice cream, frozen yogurt, ice water, and so on). The cold causes the fats in the bile to thicken and congeal. (Remember what happens to chicken soup when you put it in the refrigerator?) This is one of the many reasons Ayurveda recommends eating warm, cooked foods.

In addition, many people develop gallbladder sludge from ingesting perles of fish oils, primrose oil, flaxseed oil, and other oils rich in omega-3s and fat-soluble vitamins, such as vitamins A, D, E, and K. Dumping all this fat into the gallbladder can overwhelm its ability to break down fat. If the gallbladder holds more fat than its bile can process, a sludge will form.

In much the same way, rapid weight loss diets also contribute to sludge as the gallbladder is forced to process excessive amounts of fat too quickly. I always encourage my patients to lose weight slowly, at a rate of one to two pounds per week, and to take steps to keep their bile thinned and flowing as they lose their weight (we'll talk about those steps later in this chapter).

A buildup of sludge can lead to thickening of the bile, inflammation of the gallbladder, and gallstones, all of which can cause chronic pain under the rib cage on the right side of the body that sometimes radiates into the right shoulder or the tip of the scapula. Then there's a host of potential digestive problems, such as burping, bloating, nausea, gas, vomiting, fever, and chills, as well as complications outside the digestive tract.

It should be clear by now how important it is to keep your bile thin and flowing, allowing for proper drainage out of the gallbladder. Keep this in mind the next time you're eating a bowl of ice cream at night when your digestive fire has gone to sleep, or when you're devouring french fries while drinking an ice-cold soda.

Detecting Gallbladder Sludge

How can you detect gallbladder sludge? An ultrasound of the abdomen is the most common diagnostic tool, although sludge is often picked up through a CT scan that was ordered for something else. A HIDA scan uses radioactive material to measure gallbladder emptying, and an ERCP test uses an endoscope to place dye in the ducts of the pancreas, gallbladder, and liver to evaluate the flow through these organs.

Many patients complain of gallbladder symptoms for years, even though they don't know the origin. As with subclinical thyroid dysfunction, many diagnostic tests for the gallbladder come back normal. That's no surprise, since sludge can be difficult to diagnose. Beyond tests, there are telltale signs that your bile is not flowing. Bile darkens and turns stools brown. So pale or yellow-colored stools are a good indicator of lack of bile flow.

Proper bile flow gives you the urge to move your bowels and keeps your stools soft. With bile sludge, you can become constipated with very hard bowel movements. However, keep in mind that if you are constipated, your bowel movements will stay in the intestines for longer than normal and may then take on a dark color. In this case, the dark color is not an indicator of proper bile flow.

On the other hand, lack of bile flow can also induce diarrhea, since the bile is needed to break down fat in the intestines. When the fat is not broken down and absorbed, fatty, loose bowel movements after meals can result. You may even see droplets of fat in the toilet after a bowel movement, a sure sign that you are not digesting fats well.

Other symptoms that your bile is thick and not flowing include bloating, belching, acid reflux, nausea and vomiting, or high cholesterol. Many people with bile sludge feel that while they may not be constipated, they do not empty out completely, often having to repeatedly move their bowels throughout the day to get everything out.

Tap or press under your ribs on the right upper abdomen and see if it feels like you have any pain or a feeling of fullness, almost like a balloon is in there holding lots of water and pressing against your organs. (This is exactly what happens if bile doesn't flow because the liver produces about a quart of bile a day. Imagine the amount of distension in the gallbladder if the bile remains stuck in it.) If you have even a few of these symptoms, you can bet on the fact that your bile is much too thick.

An Ounce of Prevention to Prevent a Pound of Sludge

Medical schools cover gallbladder disease in all its manifestations: gallstones (when substances in the bile crystallize, forming stones), cholecystitis (infection of the gallbladder, usually due to a gallstone, causing pain and fever and possibly requiring surgery when infection keeps recurring), gallbladder cancer (thankfully fairly rare), and gallstone pancreatitis (when a gallstone blocks the ducts that drain the pancreas, resulting in inflammation of the pancreas).

Treatments range from gallbladder surgery to antibiotics for infection, chemotherapy and radiation for gallbladder cancer, medications to dissolve gallstones, and lithotripsy, in which high-energy shock waves are projected from a machine through the abdomen to break up the gallstones. In rare cases, a needle is used to inject chemicals directly into the gallbladder to dissolve the stones.

Despite treatment, some gallstone patients remain highly symptomatic because they are still holding on to sludge-like bile or their liver is not making enough bile.

Keep in mind, a negative gallbladder diagnostic test does not mean that your gallbladder is functioning at 100 percent. On the other hand, if you *have* been diagnosed with bile sludge or a sluggish gallbladder, there is no need to automatically assume you must have it removed. It is not that difficult to thin out the sludge so that it flows properly again. Removal of the gallbladder does not always clear up the digestive problems. In fact, sometimes it makes matters worse. However, if you have developed gallstones and you are having serious gallbladder attacks, it may be too late to assume you can reverse it at this point. In any case, whether you have it removed or not, you will still be making bile and you will still need to address the deeper issues that led to your biliary distress. Which brings us to the thyroid gland.

THE THYROID GLAND'S EFFECTS ON BILE FLOW

Several recent studies report an association between hypothyroidism (and even subclinical hypothyroidism) and problems with bile flow and gallstone formation. As it turns out, the thyroid gland can affect both bile content and bile flow.

Lack of thyroid hormones decreases the liver's metabolism of cholesterol. If the liver can't break down your cholesterol, the bile becomes supersaturated with it. In turn, that makes it difficult for the bile to flow out of the gallbladder and prevents your gallbladder muscles from contracting and emptying the bile.

Low thyroid function also decreases the secretion of bile from the liver into the gallbladder, resulting in a buildup of cholesterol crystals (which could contribute to the growth of gallstones).

And finally, low thyroid function prevents the sphincter of Oddi (the sphincter that squirts bile from the gallbladder into the duodenum) from opening, preventing bile from flowing out and allowing it to sit in the gallbladder too long, forming a thick sludge.

Let's back up and ponder this for a moment. This is one of those instances where modern research has amassed great evidence about a groundbreaking subject with huge implications for our health, yet for some reason, this information has not made its way to the patients who so sorely need it. Perhaps there is so much research that much of it goes unread?

In the early years of my practice, I was amazed by the number of patients, mostly women, but also including many men and even children, who came to my office with thyroid problems (most, but not all, subclinical). It didn't take long for me to see an association—whenever I detected thyroid problems via pulse analysis, I would always concurrently find gallbladder weakness. I noticed this combination so often that I began looking to see if there was any research to back up my findings. And there it was! These studies explained so many of my patients' overlapping symptoms: fatigue, weight gain, depression, hair loss, and arrhythmias from low thyroid function, along with constipation, high cholesterol, acid reflux, and glandular growths (fibroids, cysts, and tumors on the breasts, ovaries, and thyroid) caused by lack of bile production and flow.

WHAT HAPPENS WHEN THE BILE DOESN'T FLOW?

Reabsorption of Toxins and Hormones

When bile doesn't flow, your body retains toxins rather than eliminating them, which can be dangerous. Think of it this way: Your liver takes everything you put into your body—whether swallowed, inhaled, or absorbed through the skin—and filters it, separating out the nutrients that you need and disposing of the metabolic waste, toxins, and hormones that you do not need, carefully dumping them into the bile, which is then released into the intestines for quick removal from the body through your bowel movements. However, if the bile is too thick and unable to flow, it will remain stuck in the gallbladder, allowing toxins to reabsorb back into your body.

As you can imagine, this can have severe repercussions for your health. You end up accumulating toxins until they reach a critical mass and cause cancer or autoimmune diseases. This is why some people with good gallbladder function can be exposed to toxins year after year and not get sick, yet those with sluggish gallbladders fall ill with chronic exposure. The latter keep reabsorbing these deadly toxins, allowing them to burrow into the body, and perhaps even into the brain, leading to Parkinson's disease or other neurological disorders.

The same is true with hormones. What does estrogen do? It makes things grow; in women, it is estrogen that grows breasts and rounds out the hips at puberty. But you don't want too much growth from estrogen, so it is the job of the liver to dispose of your used estrogen by breaking it down into a water-soluble toxin and dumping it into the bile, which escorts it out of the body.

When the bile doesn't flow, your estrogen is reabsorbed, giving you high estrogen levels. Estrogen levels are meant to be in balance with progesterone levels. If estrogen becomes dominant, it can create fibroid tumors and cysts on the breasts and ovaries, and if there are a lot of other toxins circulating in your system due to, say, poor diet or alcohol use, these growths can blossom into ovarian, breast, or uterine cancers.

For women, the hormones in birth control pills, infertility drugs, and hormone replacement therapy are processed through the liver and dumped into the bile. These compounds, made from cholesterol, thicken the bile, increasing the risk of sludge formation and gallstones. Thus they tend to get stuck in the bile and are reabsorbed into the body, contributing to the high rates of uterine, breast, and ovarian cancer found in women who take these synthetic hormones.

Some of my patients who are interested in detoxification ask if they can do a liver cleanse. Invariably I tell them that we have to increase bile flow first or the cleanse will be useless. The gallbladder's role in cleansing impurities is often overlooked but crucial.

High Cholesterol

Research shows that 90 percent of patients with either clinical or subclinical hypothyroidism have high cholesterol levels. How could you not have high cholesterol if your bile can't properly break down your cholesterol or if your thyroid is preventing the liver from processing fats?

Doctors routinely write prescriptions for cholesterol-lowering statin drugs when cholesterol becomes elevated. Many nutritionists recommend that their high-cholesterol patients supplement with niacin, fish oil, and red yeast rice. However, the best approach is to address the problem of high cholesterol at its source: keep the thyroid functioning normally so the liver can process the cholesterol efficiently and keep the bile thinned out and flowing. Hundreds of our patients have lowered their cholesterol just by attending to their thyroid, liver, and gallbladder function. Again, the goal for any physician should be to fix the *reason* for the dysfunction, rather than simply treating the symptom.

Acid Reflux

As I have described, bile neutralizes the stomach acids coming into the duodenum. It also supports a natural downward flow as the digestive juices make their way through the gastrointestinal tract. This is due to the fact that bile encourages peristaltic action of the intestines, driving the food through and out of the body. If your bile isn't flowing, the acid coming into the duodenum won't be neutralized, leaving the trapped digestive juices to flow up into the esophagus, not down into the bowels, causing acid reflux. In addition, the body, in its attempts to lubricate any "channel" (esophagus) that is dry or inflamed, will produce mucus to protect the esophagus from acid damage, creating a chronic cough that won't resolve until you fix the bile flow.

The vast majority of the patients I see with acid reflux (gastroesophageal reflux disease, or GERD) are routinely given proton pump inhibitors (PPIs) to reduce stomach acid levels. This may help some patients reduce their symptoms fairly quickly, since the amount of acid in the gut can subside quickly and dramatically. However, many of my patients feel no relief or get worse because now their bile isn't flowing and on top of that they have low stomach acid from their PPIs, making it extremely difficult to digest food. Moreover, small intestinal bacterial overgrowth (SIBO) can occur in this situation because the stomach acids that squirt into the duodenum kill pathogenic bacteria coming in from the food we just ate, and now those acids have been neutralized. The latest research shows that many patients who take long-term PPIs develop SIBO.

In any case, the role of the gallbladder in causing acid reflux has been downplayed, if not overlooked. Many reflux patients will receive great benefit if they learn how to keep their bile thinned out and flowing.

Osteoporosis

If the bile doesn't flow, the pH of the digestive juices remains acid. The digestive juices are absorbed from the small intestines directly into the bloodstream, resulting in an acidic pH in the blood. Calcium will then be leached out of the bones to maintain the body's pH, leading to osteopenia and osteoporosis.

Weight Gain and Formation of Cellulite

If the fats you eat aren't sufficiently broken down by the bile, they remain stuck floating around in the bloodstream, and over time they become rancid. The body will then dump these rancid fats into the fat tissue, creating cellulite and toxic fat. (A tea of coriander seed and Indian sarsaparilla can help clean the fat tissue; see page 139.)

HOW TO KEEP YOUR BILIARY SYSTEM FUNCTIONING PROPERLY

For proper biliary function, let's outline a four-part plan:

- Promote adequate production of bile
- Keep the bile thin and moving
- Shrink small stones to ease flushing
- Flush out any bile sludge

Promote Proper Bile Production by the Liver

As stated before, first and foremost, support your thyroid function to allow the liver and gallbladder to do their jobs effectively.

In addition, one of the basic tenets of Ayurveda is to make sure that your diet includes all six tastes: sweet, sour, salty, pungent, bitter, and astringent. We tend to do this automatically as we go through the day, craving a little sweet taste here or a bitter taste there. Some foods that fall into each category:

- **Sweet:** milk, ghee, coconut, dried fruits (dates, raisins, figs, etc.), fresh sweet juicy fruits, most grains, and natural sweeteners
- **Sour:** lemons, limes, and other citrus fruits
- **Salty:** white Himalayan salt (the white variety, called *soma* salt, has a cooling effect on the liver, while the pink type contains too much agni, or heat, hence its reddish color) (see the resources section for soma salt)
- **Pungent:** black pepper, chilies, cloves, cinnamon, turmeric,

cayenne, horseradish, mustard seeds, asafoetida, and wasabi
- **Bitter:** grapefruit, limes, bitter greens (dandelion, kale, broccoli raab, escarole, radicchio, chicory, arugula, endive, etc.), cooked beet greens, and bitter melon
- **Astringent:** pomegranates, persimmons, cranberries, quinces, and, to a lesser degree, broccoli, cauliflower, artichoke, asparagus, turnips, rye, buckwheat, quinoa, apples, sprouts, and legumes

Our modern diet is primarily composed of two tastes, sweet and salty, with the other four tastes essentially missing from our palate. But a blend of all six tastes is imperative for proper digestion. The flavors of the foods you consume promote the release of digestive juices, enzymes, and bile. So strive to incorporate these six tastes in your diet throughout the day. Learn to cook with a variety of spices and fresh herbs to enhance the taste and improve your digestion of food. Food that looks and tastes great gets digested much better than dull, boring, bland food.

Though all six tastes are needed for proper digestion, it is the bitter taste that is especially good for promoting bile production in the liver. This is why many cultures recommend taking bitter herbs, such as the famous Swedish bitters, before meals. Ayurvedically speaking, problems with the liver and gallbladder are considered problems of pitta dosha being out of balance, and the bitter taste is known to pacify pitta-related disorders.

There are also many herbs and spices that promote bile production, such as chicory (found in many herbal coffee substitutes), chamomile, yellow dock, neem, guduchi, kutki (*Picrorhiza kurroa*), bhumi amla, and turmeric.

Keep Bile Thin and Moving

Avoid heavy, hard-to-digest foods such as aged cheeses, cold dairy (cold milk, ice cream, thick Greek yogurt, frozen yogurt), nut butters, red meats, deep-fried foods, and poor-quality fats such as vegetable oils, hydrogenated fats and margarines. Favor warm, cooked foods including chicken, turkey, fish, lamb, grains, vegetables, boiled milk, freshly made curd cheeses, olive oil, ghee, nuts, nut milks, seeds, and fresh as well as dried fruits.

Avoid losing weight too quickly; keep weight loss at no more than one to two pounds per week.

Focus on your food as you eat to aid your digestive processes. Look at your food when you eat it, resisting the temptation to read or divert your attention away from your meal. Your brain has a direct connection to your gut. As you look at the food, your brain can "see" what is going in, giving the gut signals to release specific types of enzymes depending on the type of food you just swallowed.

Sit quietly for about five minutes after eating to allow the digestive juices to flow and the various sphincters from the stomach, gallbladder, and pancreas to open up so they can release their contents. If you have time, after eating lie on your back for five minutes, then on your left side for five minutes, then on your right side for another five minutes. This allows the digestive organs and sphincters to relax, enabling the bile and other digestive juices to flow properly.

Chew your food well before swallowing. Digestion begins in the mouth as the enzymes in your saliva encapsulate the food. Chewing your food thoroughly will make it much easier for your digestive organs to work once you swallow the food.

Don't drink ice-cold beverages at any time of the day, but especially not when you are eating, as they put out your "digestive fire" and harden the cholesterol and fat in the bile from the food you just ate, making it very difficult to digest. Instead sip warm or room-temperature spring water throughout the day.

Don't overeat. The digestive system can only process so much food at a time. Eat moderately sized servings of food, and don't go back for seconds. A good rule of thumb to follow is to stop eating when you get that first impulse that you are full, which normally happens when your stomach is about three-fourths full. It takes about twenty minutes for your brain to register that you are indeed satiated, so it's not a good idea to eat until you are totally and utterly full.

Eat cooked foods. Cooked foods are always easier to digest than raw foods. The food has to be "cooked" by your digestive organs once it comes into the body, so you might as well make it easier to digest by cooking it before it enters the digestive tract.

Avoid birth control pills and hormone replacement therapy, which concentrate the bile, allowing for bile sludge and gallstone formation.

Avoid ingesting perles of fats, like fish oils, primrose oil, flaxseed oil, and other omega-3 oil supplements, as well as the fat-soluble vitamins, such as vitamins A, D, E, and K. They will supersaturate your bile with fat, promoting sludge formation and preventing their ultimate assimilation into the cells.

....

Cholecystokinin: Keep the Gallbladder Moving!

No, really! The word cholecystokinin literally means to "move the gallbladder." Once the stomach secretes its acidic digestive juices into the duodenum, this hormone is secreted from the duodenum, stimulating the contraction of the gallbladder and forcing it to release the bile. It also stimulates the secretion of pancreatic enzymes into the small intestine.

However, if your magnesium is low this could decrease both your gallbladder contractions (remember, magnesium relaxes the smooth muscles) and the release of cholecystokinin (CCK), resulting in decreased bile flow. And this can ultimately lead to stagnation of bile, the formation of sludge, and ultimately gallstones.

As we learned earlier (see the section on magnesium on page 54) there are many prevalent reasons for magnesium deficiency in our culture. This adds to the numerous reasons the bile may not flow and why most of us are suffering from chronic subclinical gallbladder malfunction.

....

Shrink Small Gallstones

You should not try this without supervision by an Ayurvedic practitioner, because if your stones are too large, it might be too difficult to break them down. Or if you break down a large stone and it begins to flush out through the bile ducts and isn't small enough to get through, it could block the bile duct, causing a gallbladder attack. But it is good nonetheless for you to know that we have two remedies for dissolving gallstones in our Ayurvedic pharmacopeia: pashan bhed and kulthi lentils (horse gram).

Pashan Bhed/Coleus (*Coleus forskohlii*)

Pashan bhed (its name means "stone breaker") is a well-known Ayurvedic herb that is commonly used as a lithotriptic to break up both gallstones and kidney stones. You can mix it with other herbs that support biliary function and bile production to dissolve small gallstones; see the recipe below.

In this tea, pashan bhed helps break down the stones; punarnava flushes toxins from the kidneys; kutki cleanses the liver and gallbladder, supporting healthy liver function and the proper flow of bile; triphala promotes the flow of bile out of the gallbladder; and bhumi amla cleans the liver, keeping it cool at the same time. Bhumi amla also has the unusual property of balancing excess pitta (heat) and kapha (heaviness), both of which are necessary when treating the liver and gallbladder. And finally, slippery elm binds the broken-up calcium molecules from the breakdown of the stones, aiding in their removal from the body.

ॐ Tea to Break Up Gallstones

Boil 2 cups of water for five minutes. Add 2 pinches each of crude herb powder of bhumi amla, kutki (*Picrorhiza kurroa*), pashan bhed, punarnava (*Boerhavia diffusa*), slippery elm bark, and triphala to the hot water, let steep 10 minutes, and then strain. Sip slowly over a four-hour period. Repeat daily.

Kulthi Lentils (Horse Gram)

Kulthi lentils, or horse gram, is the best remedy for breaking down gallstones and kidney stones, especially if they are not too large.

❧ Lentil "Tea" for Dissolving Gallstones (and Kidney Stones)

Boil 1 cup of spring water, and pour over a handful of kulthi lentils. Cover, and let sit on the counter in a bowl overnight. The next morning, drink the water. Refrigerate the lentils during the day with a little spring water to cover. At night, take them out of the refrigerator, strain them, then add another cup of boiled spring water, leave overnight on the counter, and drink the water in the morning. Repeat one more time, covering the lentils in water during the day in the refrigerator, straining, then soaking the lentils overnight, and drinking the water the next morning.

After drinking the water on the third day, transfer the kulthi lentils to a blender, and grind them. Then transfer them to a pot, and add enough water to cover them by about an inch, along with 1 teaspoon of ghee and 1 pinch each of coriander, cumin, fennel, and turmeric. Cook for about 30 minutes, covered, or until the ground-up lentils are soft and digestible, adding more water if necessary during the cooking process.

Make this recipe a part of your daily routine for 5 to 6 months, and then have your gallstones or kidney stones reevaluated.

Flush Out Bile Sludge

If you have been having symptoms of bile sludge (nausea, belching, vomiting, acid reflux, sluggish or too many bowel movements) and feel a fullness under the ribs on the right, the recommendations below can help your bile flow again to improve your digestion. A cautionary note: it is not recommended that you try to flush out bile sludge if you have gallstones, either large or small, since they can get stuck in a duct on their way out, creating even worse problems.

Gallbladder Release

The gallbladder is located below the ribs on the right. Lie on your left side. This allows gravity to enable the proper flow of bile out of the sphincter. Tap gently under the ribs on the right, as if you were trying to burp a baby. This will encourage the bile to flow. Periodically rub your fingers downward along the gallbladder acupuncture meridian, which runs down the sides of both legs in the area where the seam is in your pants.

Starting at the top of the thigh, over the hip area, slowly apply pressure down the meridian, from top to bottom, moving from the hip to the knee. Once you reach the knee, come back up to the hip and work out the knots and painful areas along the meridian, always moving downward, as the meridian flow moves downward.

As you work the meridian, periodically tap again on the gallbladder, going back and forth from the gallbladder tapping to running the meridian down the lateral thigh to the knee, spending extra time on areas that feel lumpy. These are the areas where the flow of prana is backed up, preventing full release of the bile.

The gallbladder meridian also runs down the back of the neck, so if your neck is stiff, work out the tight areas by rubbing down the back of the neck muscles into the upper trapezius muscles.

Finally, lie on your back and rub the gallbladder meridian down the left side of your leg several times, since the meridian runs down the left leg as well.

As you work, you may start to hear the gallbladder begin to squirt out the bile. If your stomach is very relaxed, which will aid in the sphincter opening, you will both feel and hear the bile emptying.

Keep doing this until all the bile is out, which could take up to a half hour. If you are successful, any digestive symptoms, such as nausea, will quickly disappear.

HERBS AND FOODS TO RELEASE THE BILE

Our goal here is to keep the bile flowing out of your liver and gallbladder, into your small intestine (duodenum), and downward through the rest of the small and large intestines, exiting in bowel movements. The following herbs and foods will help.

Vegetables and fruits: Eat cooked beets a few times a week. They are probably *the* best food for promoting the flow of bile out of the gallbladder. Cooked artichokes are also highly beneficial in promoting bile flow. Apples and carrots are also recommended, either eaten raw or cooked.

Herbs: Triphala, an Ayurvedic formula composed of three berries—amalaki (*Phyllanthus emblica*), bibhitaki (*Terminalia belerica*), and haritaki (*Terminalia chebula*)—is one of the best formulas to promote bile flow, lose weight, lower cholesterol, and promote normal bowel movements (decrease the dosage in cases of diarrhea and increase the dosage in cases of constipation). The tea below is also helpful.

ॐ Tea to Flush Out Bile Sludge

Boil 1 quart of water for 5 minutes, and then pour the hot water into a stainless-steel insulated thermos. Add ¼ teaspoon each of dried chicory root, whole coriander seeds, fenugreek seeds, neem, and Indian sarsaparilla root (but omit the fenugreek seeds if you have excess pitta or heat in the body). Seal the thermos, and let steep for 20 minutes, then sip slowly over the next 4 hours. Repeat daily. In addition to the herbs used here, the heat from the hot water will help melt the thick sludge.

Note: to reiterate, do not try to promote bile flow if you know you have gallstones, since you may dislodge one of them and it could get stuck in a duct and cause problems.

....

Triphala

Triphala is perhaps the most well-recognized and commonly used Ayurvedic herbal formulation. It consists of three dried and powdered fruits—amalaki, haritaki, and bibhitaki. Folklore in India says: "No mother? No worry! Triphala will take care of you just as a mother takes care of her children."

When I first began my studies of the Ayurvedic herbs I was told that sooner or later most people would develop a need for this master fruit blend. I wondered why that would be, since we have hundreds of herbs for very specific problems and there are very few formulas that everyone would need. It wasn't until I was in practice for several years that I noticed that most people developed gallbladder sludge and problems with the flow of bile not only once but several times over the course of their lives. And it turns out that triphala is excellent for promoting the flow of bile and sludge out of the gallbladder. It also helps with weight loss; lowers cholesterol; is great for sluggish digestion, gas, and bloating; relieves constipation; is balancing to all three doshas; reduces acidity in the body by allowing bile flow; prevents gallstones; scrubs the intestines of old fecal material and toxins; is great for the eyes; is a good source of vitamin C; has natural anti-inflammatory, antimicrobial, and antioxidant effects; and purifies the blood.

Now that you know all the problems that result from lack of bile flow, you can see why triphala is considered one of the most beneficial of the Ayurvedic remedies. Maybe we should reconsider the adage, "An apple a day keeps the doctor away," and replace it instead with one of the most powerful fruit-based formulas in the Ayurvedic arsenal, triphala.

THE ROLE OF FIBER

We have long known about the important role that fiber plays in our health. We have also known that people in cultures (such as ours) that have less fiber in their diet tend to suffer more serious illnesses than people in cultures with larger amounts of fiber-rich foods.

Recently, however, scientists have investigated in greater detail the role of fiber in a little-known yet critically important system in our body called enterohepatic circulation. *Entero* means "intestines" or "gut," and *hepatic* refers to the liver. The enterohepatic system is responsible for clearing all the fat-soluble waste from the bloodstream by governing the progression of bile from the liver through the small intestine and back again.

Dietary fiber is classified into two groups: insoluble and soluble. Insoluble fiber doesn't break down. It includes the fiber from wheat bran, the husk of popcorn kernels, and the skins of many fruits and vegetables. This kind of fiber acts like a broom, sweeping its way through the digestive system and adding bulk and softness to the stool.

Soluble fiber comes from structures within the cells of plants, and it absorbs water as it enters the digestive tract, dissolving into a thick, viscous gel. Both types of fiber help circulate bile through the gastrointestinal tract, but it is the soluble fiber that does most of the work.

Enterohepatic Bile Circulation

The liver produces about a quart of bile every day, which emulsifies the fats in the foods we eat, acting on the fats in much the same way that detergent breaks down grease on pots and pans. Once the food is broken down, it is absorbed in the upper part of the small intestine, known as the ileum. By the time the bile makes its way to the lower end of the small intestine (known as the terminal ileum), it has been broken down into its constituent parts, which then make their way, via the bloodstream, back to the liver to complete their journey.

At the beginning of this process, the liver is removing fats, cholesterol, fat-soluble vitamins, fat-soluble toxins, and cholesterol-based hormones from the food, medications, and supplements that we eat and dumping them into the newly created bile. At the end of the ileum the various constituents in the bile that aren't otherwise bound up pass through the intestinal wall, enter the bloodstream, and go back to the liver, where they are added to the new bile. If those constituents include toxins and xenobiotics, and this process is allowed to continue unabated, the bile will become increasingly toxic.

Here's where the benefits of fiber come in: Fiber forms a tight bond with the bile in your intestines, binding to all the harmful toxins, cholesterol, hormones, and fats. Since fiber cannot be absorbed into the intestinal wall, neither can the bile attached to it. Thus, it has no choice but to exit the body in a bowel movement, along with the toxins, cholesterol, hormones, and fats adhering to it.

This is why lack of fiber can contribute to high cholesterol and a host of other problems. Wisconsin-based nutritionist Karen Hurd, who specializes in chronic digestive disorders, notes:

> When bile is being properly escorted by fiber and carried out of the body by our stool, there are fewer bile acids recycling to the liver and being stored in the gallbladder. This means that the next time we eat a meal with fat in it, the liver has to make fresh new bile. It manufactures this new bile by pulling cholesterol (one of the key components of bile) out of the blood, thereby reducing blood cholesterol levels. Under low-fiber conditions, though, that process doesn't happen as readily and thus cholesterol has an opportunity to increase in the bloodstream, accumulating in our arteries.

She goes on to explain that as the bile becomes more toxic from reabsorbing toxins from the old bile, it becomes sludge-like, much like mud. As the bile holds on to more and more toxins, it becomes more acidic, causing inflammation in the bowel, duodenum, and even higher up into the esophagus, which can cause it to feel like the food you eat is getting stuck in your throat. It can also cause skin problems as the skin attempts to rid the body of these acidic toxins. And as these extremely sticky substances are reabsorbed back into the bloodstream, they get stuck in the arteries and clog them. Finally, she notes, the constant reabsorption of estrogen can result in numerous estrogen-type cancers, such as breast, uterine, fallopian tube, ovarian, and vaginal cancers.

The solution is easy, however: incorporate fiber-rich foods into your diet. "If you have all your fiber in one serving, it only acts on the food you eat then, not on the food you eat hours later," says Christine Gerbstadt, author of *Doctor's Detox Diet* and a spokesperson for the American Dietetic Association. "Fiber doesn't hang around waiting for the next meal. If you want fiber to bind to toxins all day, you have to eat it all day."

Adding Fiber to Your Diet

Here are some good sources of soluble fiber: beans, lentils, oat bran, oatmeal, rice bran, barley, citrus fruits, strawberries, and apple pulp.

Insoluble fiber comes from whole grains such as wheat, rye, rice, barley, and most other grains, along with cabbage, beets, carrots, brussels sprouts, turnips, cauliflower, and apple skin.

Powdered psyllium husk is excellent for binding toxins—put one teaspoon in a glass of room-temperature spring water, stir, and drink on an empty stomach. You will notice that the psyllium becomes very gelatinous and slimy as you stir it. It is this viscous quality that binds the toxins for removal from the body. Arrowroot powder, tapioca, taro root, and okra all feature this viscousness and are therefore also excellent binders to toxins. Add these items to your diet every week.

I hope that by now you can see the importance of proper liver and gallbladder function and the role the bile plays in keeping us healthy. However, I would like to add a cautionary note: While we do need fiber in our diets, we don't want to exclusively focus on fruits, vegetables, grains, and lentils to the exclusion of all other foods. In other words, we don't want to overcorrect. We are currently seeing two extremes in the Western diet. In one case, there is no fiber in the diet; these people eat only meats, cheeses, potatoes, flour products, starches, and sugary foods.

The second case is vegetarians who avoid all animal protein. Forgoing animal protein can deprive our bodies of critical nutrients. For this reason, vegetarians need to incorporate milk and milk products into their diets. On the other hand, meat eaters must make sure to eat a range of foods, including fruits, vegetables, grains, and legumes. It has become conventional wisdom but bears repeating: the best diet is a balanced one.

7

Ayurvedic Treatments
for Specific Conditions Caused
by Thyroid Dysfunction

For a gland that weighs less than an ounce, the thyroid is a task-master, performing myriad functions in our bodies. It regulates heart rhythm, controls metabolism, and contributes to our bone health, to mention only a few of its duties. So the consequences are far-reaching when the thyroid is ailing.

In the preceding chapters, we discussed techniques and remedies to address the root cause of thyroid malfunction, rebalance the immune system, and strengthen the thyroid gland. However, in some cases, even after you have taken these remedial steps, symptoms of imbalance continue. There are numerous natural remedies to address these persistent symptoms. In this chapter, we'll focus on Ayurvedic treatments for symptoms commonly seen with hypothyroidism and Hashimoto's autoimmune thyroiditis.

HAIR LOSS / BRITTLE NAILS

Bhringaraj

Bhringaraj (*Eclipta alba*) is the main herb used in Ayurveda for hair care and growth, but it maintains and rejuvenates not just the hair but also the teeth, bones, memory, sight, and hearing. It can be taken internally as well as made into an oil that is applied to the scalp. It is best to apply bhringaraj oil to the scalp and expose to the early morning sunlight (in the warmer weather) for twenty minutes to activate the follicles to grow hair.

Aloe Oil

In cases where the scalp is hot, itchy, and flaky from too much ama visha and gara visha, use of a cooling aloe oil (available from some herbal Ayurvedic companies online) is recommended. Leave the oil on for twenty minutes, then shampoo with a good-quality alkaline shampoo (free of sodium laurel sulfate, parabens, formaldehyde, petrochemicals, GMOs, phosphates, ammonia, and chlorine).

Seeds and Nuts

A sesame-almond smoothie will also encourage beautiful, lustrous hair growth; see the recipe below. Always keep in mind that the health of the hair is actually an indicator of the strength of the bones. Therefore, to have a head of thick shiny hair you must nourish the bones first and foremost. Sesame seeds contain an impressive amount of minerals necessary for maintaining bone density, such as calcium, magnesium, zinc, phosphorous, and manganese. Almonds are rich in monounsaturated fats and an excellent source of calcium and magnesium and are also very important for bone density.

Toasting and grinding the sesame seeds and soaking and peeling the almond skins allows for greatest digestion and absorption of the nutrients into the cells. The use of the spices in this formula also aids in the digestion and assimilation of the nutrients within the almonds and sesame seeds so they are absorbed adequately into the bone tissue, which will become evident in bountiful hair growth.

❧ Sesame-Almond Smoothie

10 almonds

About 1 cup whole milk, preferably organic

4 ounces toasted sesame seeds

$1/8$ teaspoon ground cardamom

$1/8$ teaspoon ground cinnamon

$1/8$ teaspoon ground cloves

$1/8$ teaspoon ground fennel seed

$1/8$ teaspoon ground ginger

$1/8$ teaspoon mace

$1/8$ teaspoon ground nutmeg

1 pinch freshly ground black pepper

Soak the almonds in water overnight, then drain, rinse, and peel. Bring the milk to a boil. Combine the almonds with the hot milk in a blender, add the remaining ingredients, and process. Drink on an empty stomach at least four times a week.

IRREGULAR HEARTBEAT / ARRHYTHMIA

Calcium and Magnesium

Calcium makes the heart contract, and magnesium makes it relax, creating a regular rhythm. When magnesium becomes depleted, the heart will beat irregularly. For these situations, we recommend transdermal use of magnesium chloride (it does not digest well when taken orally and goes through the system too quickly, producing diarrhea). In addition, we recommend bioavailable forms of calcium, such as coral calcium and a formula called *praval panchamrit,* a highly absorbable form of calcium. *Praval* means "coral" and *panch* means "five," while *amrit* qualifies this formula as a "nectar from the gods." The formula contains five sources of calcium: red coral, white coral, two types of pearls, and baby snail shells. These various sources of calcium taken from the ocean are prepared as a bhasma: they are ground up and then repeatedly incinerated, creating a fine ash whose particles are now small enough to be absorbed into the cells. Other forms of synthetic calcium supplements are not recommended since they don't absorb well into our bones and can build up in our arteries, causing plaque, hardening of the arteries, and heart attacks.

Punarnava

Punarnava (*Boerhavia diffusa*) is used to treat both hyperactive and underactive adrenal glands. It is also the primary herb used in Ayurveda to maintain proper kidney function and fluid retention.

The adrenal glands sit on top of the kidneys, producing a hormone called aldosterone. It directs our kidneys to reserve electrolytes (sodium, potassium, and others), which generate electricity, prevent fluid retention, and contract muscles, all of which are useful in maintaining a regular heart rhythm. Electrolytes are controlled by a variety of hormones, most of which are manufactured in the kidneys and adrenal glands. This makes punarnava an excellent choice in the treatment of irregular heartbeats because it supports both the kidneys and adrenal glands.

Other Herbs

Arjuna: Arjuna (*Terminalia arjuna*) has been proven to strengthen the heart muscle and is used for all types of heartbeat irregularities.

Shankhpushpi: This herb (*Convolvulus pluricaulis*) is used in Ayurveda to combat anxiety and stress, two factors in arrhythmias.

HIGH ESTROGEN/LOW PROGESTERONE

Two of the most important hormones in a woman's body are estrogen and progesterone, both of which are produced by the ovaries. Estrogen is responsible for the growth of the uterine lining during the first half of the menstrual cycle, and progesterone dominates the second half of the cycle. Progesterone, or "pro-gestation," as its name implies, prepares the uterus for implantation of fertilized eggs and pregnancy. It regulates the inner lining (endometrium) of the uterus and prevents uterine contractions that may disturb the embryo and lead to miscarriage.

There must be a balance in the ratio of estrogen to progesterone. As previously discussed, the liver takes in the used-up estrogen, breaks it down into a water-soluble toxin, and dumps it into the bile for release into bowel movements. However, when thyroid function is low, the gallbladder fails to release the bile and the estrogen can now reabsorb, creating a situation of high estrogen/low progesterone.

The most common cause of low progesterone is stress. The cortisol and adrenaline that are released by the adrenal glands during periods of high stress decrease progesterone.

To add to the problem, now we know that many of the synthetic substances we use every day mimic estrogen in the body and are even implicated in causing breast cancer. These include plastics, pesticides, herbicides, solvents, adhesives like fingernail polish, cleaning supplies, automobile exhaust fumes, and polychlorinated biphenyls (PCBs). PCBs, man-made chemicals that were once used in producing electrical equipment, surface coatings, inks, adhesives, flame retardants, and paints, are banned today, but about 10 percent of the PCBs produced since 1929 still remain in the environment today.

Excess estrogen can stimulate uterine bleeding and result in long menstrual cycles, midcycle bleeding, menstrual cycles coming every two weeks, or nonending menstrual cycles, sometimes going on for a month or more. It can also cause fibroids in the uterus and cysts in the breasts or ovaries.

Three herbs are commonly used to rebalance the ratio between estrogen and progesterone: lodhra (*Symplocos racemosa*), ashoka (*Saraca asoca*), and coriander (*Coriandrum sativum*). The tea recipe below uses all three in combination and is excellent for midcycle bleeding or heavy bleeding and long menstrual cycles in general.

❧ Tea for Heavy Menstrual Bleeding

Boil 1 quart of water for 5 minutes, and then pour the hot water into a stainless-steel insulated thermos. Add ¹/₂ teaspoon each of lodhra, ashoka, and whole (not ground) coriander seed. Seal the thermos, and let steep for 20 minutes, then sip slowly over the next 4 hours.

Repeat daily. If menstrual bleeding remains excessive after a few days on this tea, add ¹/₂ teaspoon of white oak bark to stem the bleeding. If you are bleeding heavily due to fibroids or ovarian cysts, add $^1/_2$ teaspoon of kanchanar powder as well. Kanchanar is famous for shrinking glandular growths, such as cysts on breasts and ovaries, thyroid nodules, and uterine fibroids.

This recipe works very quickly and has saved many women from having to take birth control pills or progesterone due to heavy bleeding.

One final note: avoid eating fennel bulb and drinking fennel seed tea, as fennel is highly estrogenic and will work against you in your efforts to rebalance the ratio of estrogen to progesterone. Asparagus, pineapple, and papaya are also estrogenic (to a much lesser extent than fennel) and should be reduced in the diet—you may still consume them, but don't have them more than two or three times a week.

DEPRESSION

Arjuna

This herb is widely used as a heart tonic and is perhaps the best herb to counteract emotional stress. It is especially effective when combined with rose petals, which are used as a treatment for sadness and emotional turmoil.

Ashoka

This herb, whose name means "without sorrow" or "no grief," is especially helpful for anyone grieving the death of a loved one. In addition, it has the side benefit of preventing heavy menstrual bleeding due to its tonic effects on the uterus.

Mucuna

We recommend mucuna (*Mucuna pruriens*) for patients whose depression is accompanied by low energy and lack of motivation. It has been used for centuries to balance the reproductive and nervous systems, increasing libido in both men and women. It is one of the best food sources of the amino acid L-dopa, a direct precursor to the neurotransmitter dopamine, which improves mood and increases energy.

WEIGHT GAIN

Shilajit (mineral pitch)

Shilajit is perhaps the best herb for weight loss. According to Ayurveda, shilajit possesses *lekhaniya,* or fat-scraping qualities that remove excess fat in the body. This remedy helps you burn off calories rather than converting them into fat. A cautionary note, however: because this remedy burns fat, it is capable of creating excess heat in the liver, so it is best used as part of a formula with other herbs that can balance its heating qualities, rather than on its own. There are dozens of formulas with shilajit available from herbal Ayurvedic companies online.

Garcinia

Garcinia (*Garcinia cambogia*) is a tropical fruit that contains hydroxy-citric acid (HCA), which is known to suppress appetite and prevent fat production. HCA works by preventing an enzyme, citrate lyase, from working. Citrate lyase converts carbohydrates into fats that are then stored in the body.

You can buy garcinia capsules or make a tea. Here's one of many recipes.

ॐ Garcinia Tea

Boil 1 quart of water for 5 minutes, and then pour the hot water into a stainless-steel insulated thermos. Add ¹/₂ teaspoon of garcinia, 2 whole green cardamom pods, a ¹/₂-inch piece of cinnamon stick, and 1 whole black peppercorn. Seal the thermos, and let steep for 20 minutes, then sip slowly over the next 4 hours.

Betel Leaf

Chewing betel leaves after a meal to freshen the mouth is a very common Ayurvedic practice. Betel leaf is also a great weight loss tool. Studies have shown that it speeds up metabolism, and according to the ancient Ayurvedic texts, the leaves help reduce meda dhatu (fat tissue), hastening weight loss. When combined with kulthi lentils, they become a powerful tool to reduce body fat.

Kulthi Lentils

Kulthi lentils grow on hard rocky soil in the Himalayas, and it is said that, being hardy enough to grow on rocks, they have the intelligence to break up calcifications. They are used primarily to break up kidney stones and calcified toxins, and they have a side benefit of enhancing weight loss by helping to scrape away fat tissue.

Kulthi lentils are available in most Indian grocery stores; they are sometimes called horse gram. They are prepared by being boiled in water with spices, vegetables, and ghee, just like a lentil soup. However, they need to be finely ground for a few minutes in a blender before use because they are as hard as rocks and take hours to cook otherwise. When ground, they will cook in 30 to 40 minutes.

Fenugreek and Cumin

Fenugreek enhances fat (and sugar) metabolism, and cumin reduces kapha, or heaviness, in the body. You can cook with these spices, but since they have a fat-burning capability, be careful if you have excess heat (pitta) in your body or suffer from excess liver heat.

Dietary Considerations

In addition to the herbs noted above, it is important to avoid wheat and rice, the two heaviest grains. The ancient doctors said that if you want to lose weight, eat barley every other day, as barley is the most kapha-reducing grain. (However, barley contains gluten; if you are on a gluten-free diet, try lighter grains such as millet, buckwheat, oats, quinoa, or amaranth instead.)

Even if you tend to gain weight easily, whole milk is still preferable to the highly processed low-fat and skim milks. If you want to reduce your milk calories, use a dilution of half whole milk and half water when making oatmeal or other hot cereals.

Be sure to include ghee in your diet. Eliminating or limiting fats will leave you hungry and prone to binging. Through the years I have watched many people lose weight by adding ghee and boiled whole milk to their diets. Ghee from grass-fed cows contains conjugated linoleic acid (CLA), which can lower body fat! Whole milk and ghee are excellent for pacifying the appetite control centers in the brain because of their satiating and nourishing qualities.

OSTEOPENIA OR OSTEOPOROSIS

As we have discussed in previous chapters, thyroid hormones play a pivotal role in bone metabolism. I see many patients with thyroid problems and associated gallbladder malfunction diagnosed with osteopenia or osteoporosis. It is treatable in the early stages, so it is best you follow these guidelines as soon as you see your bones are thinning. In addition to keeping your thyroid and gallbladder in good working condition, add this to your overall program to keep up your bone strength as you age.

Following are the nutrients needed for good bone health, and the best sources of those nutrients. Please do keep in mind, however, that the minerals mentioned here have to adhere to a matrix of collagen. Collagen is found in animal protein, so it is of utmost importance you keep up your protein intake or all the calcium and magnesium in the world will not be able to increase your bone density (see dietary recommendations for protein sources listed in chapter 8, page 171, and the bone broth information on page 107 for good sources of collagen).

Calcium
Seniors are advised to consume at least 1,000 to 1,200 milligrams of calcium a day. However, when a person takes a calcium supplement and you take their pulse, you can feel the calcium stuck in their bloodstream. In other words, calcium supplements are not absorbed into the bone cells. Even worse, unabsorbed calcium can clog artery walls, attaching to areas where oxidized fats lie, contributing to plaque formation and hardening of the arteries. In fact, researchers have found no proof that

boosting calcium intake beyond normal dietary levels strengthens bones or prevents fractures.

"We've gathered all the clinical studies of calcium supplements and dietary calcium intake for both bone density and fractures," wrote M. Bolland et al., a team of researchers in New Zealand. "Taken together, we think this is the strongest possible evidence that taking calcium supplements will not be beneficial. Moreover, excess calcium supplementation can be harmful."

Clinical trials have shown that calcium supplements often cause minor gastrointestinal side effects and increase the risk of kidney stones, heart attacks, and joint pain. Side effects such as these are typical from synthetic nutraceuticals.

It is best to get your calcium from a natural source, such as coral calcium or praval panchamrit (both discussed as useful supplements for irregular heartbeat earlier in this chapter). Don't forget that good-quality milk, as long as it is not consumed cold, is perhaps the best source of calcium in the diet. Soft-curd cheeses, such as ricotta, fresh mozzarella, cottage cheese, farmer's cheese, and paneer, as well as home-made yogurt, are also excellent sources of calcium.

Magnesium

In her book *The Magnesium Miracle,* Carolyn Dean, M.D., N.D., notes the importance of magnesium in the prevention and treatment of osteoporosis. Bones need both calcium and magnesium, she explains. Calcium makes bones hard, but like a piece of chalk, if you drop it, it will break. Magnesium makes the bones pliable, like a chicken bone, which you can bend without breaking.

In my practice, we recommend transdermal magnesium therapy. There are several excellent transdermal magnesium products on the market that contain magnesium chloride, which is the best form to use. Some practitioners recommend Epsom salts, but they contain magnesium sulfate, which the body must convert to the chloride form, so it is best to use magnesium chloride in the first place. Plus, magnesium sulfate has a short-lived response compared to the longer-acting chloride form.

That said, look carefully for pure magnesium products, as the lakes and seas from which these magnesium salts are sourced are often contaminated with heavy metals, such as mercury and lead, from coal plant emissions. This is why we recommend magnesium from an ancient seabed in the Zechstein Sea, which is located 250 miles below the surface of the Earth, where it remains free from the effects of air pollution. Its salts have been tested and found to contain no traces of lead or mercury.

Vitamin D

Vitamin D is the name of a group of fat-soluble secosteroids, cholecalciferol (vitamin D_3) and ergocalciferol (vitamin D_2). Vitamin D_3 is produced in our skin after exposure to ultraviolet B (UVB) light from the sun, and both vitamins D_2 and D_3 occur naturally in fish (including cod liver oil) and eggs. However, as discussed in earlier chapters, it is nearly impossible to get adequate amounts of vitamin D from your diet. Sunlight exposure is the only reliable way to generate vitamin D in your body.

Sufficient levels of vitamin D are crucial for calcium absorption in your intestines, which maintains the health of your bones and teeth. You can take supplements of vitamin D, but as with most nutraceuticals, there are side effects, and for vitamin D in particular, there is no consensus on the optimal dose. In 2010 the National Institutes of Health set the recommended dietary allowance (RDA) at 600 IUs daily for infants, children, and adults up to seventy years of age. This was an increase from their previous recommendation of 200 IUs daily. However, as we have pointed out, the body does not tend to process synthetic supplements very well, and those nutraceuticals can build up in the body over time, leading to toxicity. We just don't have solid scientific evidence about the long-term safety of high doses of vitamin D supplementation.

Nevertheless, many people I see have low levels of vitamin D even if they live in areas with abundant sunshine and spend a lot of time in the sun. So we want to look deeper into the issue to see *why* so many of us have low levels of vitamin D. Research points to the primary cause being high calcium levels, which suppress vitamin D production. There are several possible causes of high calcium levels:

- Regular use of synthetic calcium
- Magnesium deficiency (very common)
- Acidic pH (also very common in a culture with a highly processed diet)
- Protein deficiency
- Liver dysfunction
- Vitamin K_2 deficiency (this vitamin ensures the proper use of calcium in your body; see below)

When vitamin D supplementation is called for, we recommend transdermal vitamin D derived from cod liver oil. Transdermal application is preferred because vitamin D, a fatty vitamin, can supersaturate your bile over time and create gallbladder sludge. You cannot overdose with transdermals; your body will simply take what it needs, saving you from the potentially serious consequences of the very real prospect of overdosing when taking oral supplements.

Vitamin K_2

There are four fat-soluble vitamins: A, D, E, and K. Vitamins A, D, and E are stored in your body fat, but vitamin K is not, so deficiency is common.

Vitamin K_2 directs calcium away from your arteries and into your bones. In so doing, it prevents dangerous calcium deposits in the arteries and osteoporosis.

Vitamin K_2 is extremely rare in our diets. It is, however, found in ghee made from the milk of grass-fed cows.

Asthi Shrinkala

Asthi shrinkala (*Cissus quadrangular*) nourishes and detoxifies the bone tissue. It is widely used in Ayurveda to increase bone mass and can even accelerate the healing of fractures.

You can buy asthi shrinkala in capsule form, taking one after breakfast and one after dinner, or prepare it as a daily tea: stir ½ teaspoon of the powdered herb into a large mug of hot water, let steep for ten minutes, and sip slowly.

Guduchi

Guduchi satwa (*Tinospora cordifolia*) is made from juicing the starchy stem of the guduchi plant and drying it into a powder. This unique herb has the capability of reaching the bone marrow and can clean it and reduce inflammation at this very deep level of the bone, where the bone cells, the osteoblasts and osteoclasts, are made. The osteoblasts build up the bone tissue, while the osteoclasts are responsible for breaking down the bone. Thus, the bone tissue is constantly in a state of flux, breaking down old bone and restoring it with new healthy bones.

However, if there are toxins or inflammation in the bone marrow, the stem cells there divert and mistakenly increase their production of the osteoclasts, causing too much breakdown of the bone, which can lead to osteopenia and osteoporosis.

This is yet one more example of the far-reaching and multiple uses of guduchi satwa, which is why the ancient seers considered this one of the most beneficial herbs for protecting our health. Keep in mind it is the bone marrow where both the immune system *and* the bone cells are born. Therefore this very distinctive herb can be a powerful tool in the treatment of autoimmune diseases, cancer, and osteoporosis, all problems arising from toxins sitting in the bone marrow.

HIGH CHOLESTEROL

As explained previously, when the thyroid gland malfunctions, the sphincter of Oddi, found in the gallbladder, has trouble releasing bile. Bile contains detergent-like compounds that emulsify dietary fats into very small droplets for absorption and assimilation into cells. When the thyroid is weak and bile doesn't flow, your cholesterol levels can increase as these fats are left free to circulate in your blood rather than being absorbed into cells to be burned up and converted into energy.

Ayurveda uses numerous herbs to promote bile flow. I generally recommend the ones described below.

Triphala

As stated previously triphala is a popular Ayurvedic formula consisting of three fruits—haritaki, amalaki, and bibhitaki—whose properties are balancing to all three body types, vata, pitta, and kapha respectively. The combination of the three fruits works together, providing a variety of health benefits. It is a natural antioxidant, boosts the immune system, and nourishes and rejuvenates tissues.

It maintains regularity and naturally cleanses and tonifies the bowel. Among other things, it is a great tonic for the gallbladder, as it promotes bile release. As bile begins to flow, triphala can increase the urge in some people to move their bowels.

You can drink it as a tea or take it as a tablet either at bedtime or after meals. Cut back on the dose if it creates too many bowel movements. Conversely increase the dose if you are still constipated on a low dose.

Neem

Neem (*Azadirachta indica*) is a famous Ayurvedic herb used primarily for skin conditions because it cleans oily, acne-prone skin and contains antifungal and antibacterial properties. Its extremely bitter taste cleans the liver and encourages bile flow, both of which are needed to keep cholesterol levels down. This herb contains a little heat, so cut down on it if you feel any burning in your stomach.

Indian Sarsaparilla

This herb aids in the digestion and elimination of fats, thus helping to lower cholesterol circulating in the bloodstream. When the bile isn't flowing, the fats in the diet won't be absorbed into your cells and therefore will remain stuck in the bloodstream (which is why the cholesterol will go up) and intestines, going rancid. The body, in attempts to rid itself of these rancid fats, will dump them into the fat cells, creating toxic fat tissue (meda dhatu). Indian sarsaparilla (*Hemidesmus indicus*) is the best herb to clean the fat tissue.

This herb is also indicated when your fats aren't digesting and absorbing properly and are instead dumped into your bowel movement, where you will notice little globules of fat. This is the best herb used to treat this condition. This herb is unique in that even though it helps to burn fats and cholesterol it still has a cooling property and can be used when there is excess pitta in the body (unlike neem and fenugreek).

Fenugreek Seeds

Research has shown the efficacy of fenugreek seeds, sometimes called *methi,* in our diets (or in tea) to lower cholesterol. However, since they have a heating tendency, we recommend that you use them sparingly if you know you have an excess pitta condition.

ॐ Tea to Lower Cholesterol

Boil 1 quart of water for 5 minutes, and then pour the hot water into a stainless-steel insulated thermos. Add ¼ teaspoon each of whole coriander seeds, fenugreek seeds, neem, and Indian sarsaparilla root. Seal the thermos, and let steep for 20 minutes, then sip slowly over the next 4 hours.

This tea works to not only lower cholesterol but also cleanses the liver, blood, and fat tissue.

Guduchi

Due to its ability to cleanse the liver and support liver function, guduchi leaves and stems are commonly used in Ayurvedic practice for lowering cholesterol. The leaves can be heating, though, so it is best to avoid that part of the plant if you suffer from excess pitta or symptoms of excess heat, such as headaches, rashes, or loose bowels, to name just a few. Instead, use the plant's starchy stem (guduchi sattwa).

If you take plain guduchi tablets, one tablet after breakfast and one after dinner is the recommended dose. If you are able to obtain guduchi sattwa powder, stir ¼ teaspoon into ¼ cup of room-temperature spring water and drink after meals, two or three times a day.

CONSTIPATION

There are many reasons for constipation:

Lack of bile flow due to thyroid weakness: Use triphala or haritaki, which can stimulate bile flow and thus loosen the bowels. Triphala and haritaki are not considered laxatives and thus are not addicting like senna and cascara sagrada, well-known herbal laxatives that are contraindicated.

Vata disturbance: Since the seat of vata lies in the apana region, home to our intestines, and vata is the element of air and dryness, sometimes our digestive tracts become too dry, which causes constipation. Try boiling a cup of milk and adding a teaspoon of ghee. Sip this slowly in the evening to lubricate your bowels the next day.

Dehydration: Drink plenty of pure alkaline spring water, sipping it slowly throughout the day. Do not drink too much before, during, or after meals; too much water can dilute your digestive enzymes.

Certain foods are indicated in the treatment of constipation: cooked prunes, okra, beets, blueberries, mangoes, cooked cabbage, and sweet juicy pears. Try these foods to see if they work for you. Always eat fresh fruits in between meals on an empty stomach as they digest rapidly and may ferment in the stomach while waiting for other foods to be digested.

Dried fruits, such as prunes, should either be soaked overnight in a bowl of spring water on the counter or cooked, to reconstitute them with water. You always want to avoid dried foods as they will create a dry bowel movement. This includes both dried fruits and drying foods such as rice cakes, pretzels, and crackers. Also avoid too many grains, pastas, and breads, as they are binding as well. (Remember, vata is the element of dryness, so too many dry foods will constipate you.)

INSOMNIA AND ANXIETY

Most of the remedies for calming the mind can be used interchangeably for addressing both insomnia and anxiety.

Ashwagandha

One of the best herbs for treating the thyroid gland, ashwagandha prevents the release of too much cortisol from the adrenal glands when we are under stress, which can create problems with falling or staying asleep. In addition, ashwagandha's sedative effect encourages restful sleep, and it is therefore used in many of the Ayurvedic sleep formulas.

Boiled Milk with Spices

Combine a cup of milk with a pinch each of cardamom, cinnamon, nutmeg, and turmeric. Boil the milk with these spices for three minutes, then strain (if you used whole spices), and sip slowly before bedtime. This will induce sleep and help you sleep through the night.

Calamus Root

Calamus root is a natural sedative that is commonly used to calm the nerves and relieve insomnia.

Jatamansi

Jatamansi (*Nardostachys jatamansi*) balances brain neurotransmitters and aids sleep. A strong sedative and tranquilizer, it is related to valerian and can calm down overstimulation of the mind, promoting deep sleep. This wonderful herb is a better remedy for insomnia than melatonin supplements. Your pineal gland makes melatonin; if you take it orally, your own pineal gland will promptly shut down its production. A good rule of thumb is to not take anything your body already makes but instead to help your body heal so that it can produce that substance on its own.

Valerian Root

Used by both Ayurvedic and Western practitioners, valerian root (*Valeriana officinalis*) promotes relaxation and sleep and decreases stress. It helps you fall asleep faster, provides a better sleep quality, and provides relief from restlessness and other anxiety-related symptoms.

White Poppy Seeds

Less well known than black sesame seeds, these seeds can pacify vata in the mind (prana vata). When the mind is overactive, it can interfere with good-quality sleep. You can add white poppy seeds to your grains and oatmeal during the day, or try a batch of white poppy seed chutney (see the recipe below) right before bed.

ॐ White Poppy Seed Chutney

Mix 1 teaspoon of white poppy seeds with 1 teaspoon of coconut (shredded fresh coconut is best, but dried is fine). Melt $\frac{1}{2}$ teaspoon of ghee in a small pan over medium heat until it becomes clear, then add a pinch each of ground cumin and ground turmeric. Remove from heat immediately, add to the poppy seed mixture, and mix well. Let stand for 5 minutes, then add a pinch of salt and eat.

Note: White poppy seeds contain small quantities of psychoactive opiates, primarily morphine. Research shows that morphine and codeine can sometimes be detected in the urine up to 48 hours after ingestion of poppy seeds, so you may want to forgo the use of poppy seeds if you must undergo urine drug tests at your workplace or for any other reason.

Oil Treatments

Abhyanga

Abhyanga, or daily oil massage, is often recommended for detoxification and for nourishing and rejuvenating the body and mind, and it is also a wonderful remedy for anxiety and insomnia. See page 48 for instructions. For treating anxiety and insomnia in particular, you might look for a vata-balancing oil, which will further calm the nerves. Rubbing a vata-balancing oil into your scalp and/or the soles of your feet is also highly effective in the treatment of insomnia.

Nasya

Nasya is the practice of administering a medicinal oil through the nasal passages. As noted in chapter 1, the nostrils are a channel through which prana enters the body, which is why the nostrils are called the "gateways to the head" (*shirodwar*) in Sanskrit. Nasya is used to keep open these very important pathways, allowing the unimpeded flow of prana into our bodies.

Nasya oils are infused with healing herbs and used to nurture, nourish, and calm the mind, lubricate and cleanse the nasal passages, and so much more, depending on the herbs that are used. Most Ayurvedic herbal companies offer various types of nasya oils. For relief from anxiety and insomnia, try the ones infused with two species of brahmi (which are gotu kola and *Bacopa monneiri*), as well as skullcap, jatamansi, calamus root, and other calming herbs. Place three to five drops of the oil in each nostril, use a finger to rub the oil into the inner walls of the nasal passages, then sniff or snort it in. Rest for a few minutes while lying on your back to allow the oil to sink in.

Shirodhara

Shirodhara, whose name derives from the Sanskrit *shiro* (head) and *dhara* (flow), is a traditional Ayurvedic technique that involves pouring warmed medicinal oil (such as sesame and others infused with vata-pacifying herbs) over the *ajna* or *sthapani marma,* the area in between the eyebrows, which has direct effects on the nervous system. As the oil penetrates into your nerves, you can experience a profound state of rest, similar to a deep meditation.

Marma points are the combination of all three aspects of prana: soma, agni, and marut. As noted earlier, these points can be activated to supply prana to specific organs, glands, systems, and spirit.

The ajna marma point is considered one of the very powerful energy centers of the body. Pouring a continuous flow of warm oil on this point can enhance cerebral circulation, allowing for optimal functioning of the pituitary and pineal glands, which improves concentration and memory, balances the emotions, and calms the mind, promoting deep and restful sleep.

Ayurveda especially recommends shirodhara for rebalancing vata, which can present as fear, insecurity, worry, and racing thoughts, and pitta, which can cause anger, irritability, frustration, and judgment.

You will have to seek out a qualified Ayurvedic practitioner for a shirodhara treatment.

JOINT PAIN

Vitiated (out of balance) vata is the major cause of both thyroid problems and joint and bone pain. Always remember to keep vata balanced through a healthy diet and early bedtime, avoiding stress whenever possible; see page 11 for more details.

Joint stiffness and pain also occur from ama settling in the joints. As you'll recall, ama is produced when food is heavy and hard to digest; see page 64 for more details. So make sure your diet is both nutritious and easy to digest, meaning that you should favor warm, cooked meals over cold, raw foods. Periodic cleanses will eliminate the ama stuck in joints. You can also try the following remedies.

Boswellia

The *Boswellia serrata* tree produces a resin, also called frankincense, that acts similarly to steroids like prednisone. Boswellia can decrease pain and improve mobility in painful joints in as little as a week or two. Because of its outstanding anti-inflammatory capabilities, it is also used to treat diarrhea, bronchitis, asthma, cough, hemorrhoids, and inflammatory bowel disease. It is so safe that it can be used throughout pregnancy.

Mahanarayan Oil

This ancient herbal formula is used in abhyanga massage in the treatment of sore and stiff joints. It delivers powerful herbs used for treating muscles and joints infused in sesame oil. Both the herbs and oil will absorb directly into the affected joints and muscles, both healing and lubricating the painful areas. In addition to mahanarayan oil, many of the Ayurvedic herbal companies have varying types of herbalized oils and transdermal creams used for relieving joint and muscle pain.

Nirgundi

Nirgundi (*Vitex negundo*) is perhaps the best herb to effectively heal both the cartilage in the joints and discs in the spine. It also reduces pain and inflammation of the muscles and the joints. I can easily attest to the tremendous healing properties of this herb. Of all the herbs I use to treat joint pain, this one seems to alleviate the pain the quickest, and it not only relieves the pain but actually heals the cartilage and joints so that the effects are seen for years after discontinuing the herb.

Shringa Bhasma

This remedy is prepared from deer antler velvet, which is ground and then repeatedly incinerated to make a bhasma. Containing calcium, zinc, magnesium, and some amino acids, shringa bhasma is primarily used for the treatment of respiratory disorders such as coughs, wheezing, chest congestion, and chest tightness; it is great for bronchitis, pneumonia, and coughs due to colds.

However, like many herbal remedies, shringa bhasma has a side benefit (as opposed to pharmaceuticals, which have side effects!). The benefit is that it works wonders to heal the cartilage in our discs and joints, being especially useful for bulging discs and osteoarthritis. Many of my patients have received quick and lasting relief of joint pain from shringa bhasma.

Yoga

Most forms of gentle stretching, and especially yoga, are great for joint pain, allowing the flow of prana through the body and aiding in the elimination and movement of toxins from joints.

RESTLESS LEGS SYNDROME

Restless legs syndrome (RLS) is a nervous disorder causing uncomfortable and unpleasant sensations in the legs, worsening during periods of rest or inactivity, such as lying or sitting. These unpleasant sensations are relieved by movements such as walking or stretching. The symptoms of RLS usually occur during the evening or night.

Neurologists have always related RLS to a dysfunction in the neurotransmitter dopamine, a chemical used by brain cells to communicate and produce smooth muscle activity and movement. Decreased levels of dopamine disrupt these neurochemical signals to the muscles, creating involuntary movements.

The latest research has shown that iron insufficiency is the single most consistent finding and the strongest risk factor associated with RLS. Low iron levels when combined with hyperthyroidism—high thyroid hormone or TSH—during periods of stress contribute greatly to restless leg syndrome.

Yet only about 15 percent of the RLS population shows an iron deficiency in blood work. This led investigators to discover that the brain can be deficient in iron even if the blood work shows normal serum iron levels, as proven by cerebrospinal fluid analysis obtained by lumbar puncture. MRI studies and studies from the RLS Foundation brain bank (where RLS patients donate their brains for study) have also shown low iron in the substantial nigra, the area of the brain where dopamine is produced, and iron deficiency in the dopamine-producing cells.

There are still gaps in the knowledge, and researchers hope to figure out exactly how the brain can be low in iron while other parts of the body have normal levels.

The rhythm of symptoms for a patient who suffers from RLS follow the rhythm of thyroid-stimulating hormone (TSH) release. Thus, as levels of TSH increase in the evening, so does the severity of RLS symptoms. We now know that dopamine inhibits TSH secretion, and it also breaks down thyroid hormones. The enzymes that accomplish both these tasks are based on iron. Thus, if iron levels become depleted, then thyroid hormone can build up and so can TSH, causing RLS. To date, therapies that can increase dopamine production have been considered to be the best therapy for RLS disturbances.

We have our RLS patients consume iron-rich foods like Black Mission figs, Medjool dates, raisins, prunes, blackstrap molasses, cooked greens, and cooked beets. If a patient's iron levels are extremely low, we give iron bhasma.

We also give RLS patients mucuna, an herb that has dopamine-like qualities without the side effects of synthetically made dopamine. In addition, we have our patients rub their legs with transdermal magnesium creams or oils before bed, which helps with proper nerve firing and conduction.

8

Diet and Daily Routine
for Thyroid Health

The doctor of the future will give no medicine but will interest his patients in the care of the human frame, in the diet, and in the cause and prevention of disease.

THOMAS EDISON

The shastras, the ancient texts of Ayurveda, state that the first steps toward ill health begin with poor diet and daily routine. So to prevent any disease, we first and foremost recommend a healthy diet and early bedtime in our treatment protocols.

Proper diet is extremely important to the proper function of your thyroid. Malnourishment, whether from insufficient food or poor-quality food, will prevent you from both making and using thyroid hormone. The thyroid is also very sensitive to stress of any kind: it wilts when you work too many hours, overexercise at the gym, or stay up late binge-watching your favorite Netflix series.

There are many stressors we can't control—accidents and injuries, bills to be paid, job interviews, the never-ending chores that leave you no time left in the day to just sit and unwind. However, I always give my patients this advice: control what you can, which is primarily your diet and daily routine. If you can keep a reasonably healthy diet, following roughly 80 percent of the guidelines I lay out, allowing the occasional hot fudge sundae or chocolate chip cookie raid, and if you can make a commitment to go to bed no later than 10 p.m., your thyroid will thank you the next time you face an onslaught of stress—like when your dog gets sprayed by a skunk, requiring numerous baths in tomato juice, and your eight-year-old comes home with head lice.

Heeding these guidelines will give you a solid foundation, making it more difficult for the body to fall out of balance. Many of the patients I have seen through the years who eat healthfully and go to bed early exhibit robust health, whereas those who do not eat nutritious food or go to sleep in the wee hours of the morning always complain of fatigue and numerous other symptoms.

DIGESTION FROM THE AYURVEDIC PERSPECTIVE: A QUICK REVIEW

As we have discussed in greater detail earlier in this book, once we swallow food, it travels through a physical channel: the esophagus, stomach, small and large intestines, and out through the rectum and anus. As the food is traveling through this channel, it needs to be broken down into smaller and smaller particles so that it can eventually travel through the delicate cell walls and into the cells. Once the food is properly digested and assimilated, you should feel light, buoyant, satisfied, and refreshed with energy and bliss.

If, however, the food doesn't fully break down, it can remain stuck in the channel, forming ama. As the food sits, it starts to ferment and form acid toxins, resulting in ama visha. These acidic toxins contribute to inflammation, which is at the root of cancer and autoimmune diseases, among other diseases.

Once food is properly digested and absorbed out of the digestive system, it enters the blood and goes through various physical channels (arteries, veins, arterioles, capillaries), and then it is transformed to become part of urine (passing through the kidney tubules, ureters, and bladder), sweat (going through the sweat pores), lymph (passing through lymph vessels), and breath (going through the lung channels or bronchial tubes), among other things. The point is, once you swallow food, it ultimately makes its way through thousands of microchannels. The ancient doctors said that there were so many channels they couldn't possibly be counted.

Several things can happen to these channels: they can shrink, get clogged, or become inflamed, all of which prevents their normal flow. When flow is obstructed, illness begins. Thus, we ask our patients to avoid foods that shrink, clog, and inflame the channels.

FOODS TO AVOID

The following foods tend to shrink, clog, and inflame the channels of the body.

Nightshades: Nightshade vegetables contain nicotine, which shrinks the channels. Avoid eggplant, bell peppers (small chilies are okay), tomatoes, and white potatoes (sweet potatoes and yams are allowed).

Onions and garlic: Onions and garlic act like antibiotics in the body, and their long-term use can deplete the friendly gut bacteria and lay the foundation for food allergies and autoimmune diseases.

Vinegar: Vinegar is too acidic and sour for ingestion. Use freshly squeezed lime juice instead—it has a sour taste but turns alkaline quickly. Lemon can be used as well, but it takes longer to turn alkaline.

Seeds: Avoid chia, hemp, and pumpkin seeds, which are channel clogging. Other kinds of seeds are fine to eat; see page 188 for more details.

Red meat, pork, and processed meat: Avoid beef, pork (including ham, sausage, and bacon), and other red meats, as well as all processed meat products.

Mushrooms: Mushrooms are channel clogging and are best avoided in the diet.

Winter squashes: Avoid all winter squashes (including acorn squash, butternut squash, spaghetti squash, and pumpkin) as they are channel clogging.

Hard aged cheeses: American cheese, cheddar, Colby/Jack, Edam, blue cheese, Gorgonzola, Brie, Gouda, Camembert, provolone, Asiago, feta, cotija, Gruyere, Monterey Jack, Havarti, Stilton, Taleggio, Swiss, Boursin, fontina, Roquefort, Emmental, Jarlsberg, pepper jack, Muenster, and many other cheeses that have been aged and have lost their water content clog the channels.

Soy products: Avoid all unfermented soy products—including tofu, edamame, and soy milk—as the fat in the soybean cannot cross the delicate cell walls and will therefore clog the channels.

Large beans: These include kidney beans, cannellini beans, black beans, chickpeas (including hummus), and pinto beans. These large beans are somewhat heavy and hard to digest, which accounts for the gas experienced by those who consume them. Gas is formed as the food sits stuck in the intestines (or channels) and begins to ferment and form toxins.

Nut butters: Most nuts are fine to eat (see page 188), but avoid nut butters, like peanut butter, almond butter, and cashew butter. Nut milks, such as almond and cashew milk, are easier to digest and absorb. Notice how difficult it is to swallow a nut butter, like almond butter. And the throat is one of the largest channels in the body! Now think how clogged up the smaller delicate microchannels become as these heavy nut butters course through them.

Tahini: Also avoid tahini. While it is more thinned out than a nut butter it is still considered channel clogging. The best way to consume sesame seeds is to dry toast, then grind them for best absorption in the cells. Sprinkle on salad dressings, oatmeal, grains, and other foods.

Cold dairy products: Cold dairy clogs the channels. Avoid cold milk, ice cream, frozen yogurt, and so on. There is a lot of fat in dairy products, which congeals when it is cold. This is why Ayurveda recommends cooking and heating dairy products: boiling milk, melting fresh mozzarella cheese, baking ricotta cheese in the oven, and generally adding heat to any dairy product will make it more digestible as the cooking process breaks down the heavy fat in the milk product.

WHAT CAN I EAT?

Best Sources of Protein

Try chicken, turkey, fish, lamb, and rabbit. For nonanimal protein sources, favor the smaller lentils, such as green lentils, French lentils, and dahls (split mung dahl and red lentils), over the larger beans listed above.

Grains

Avoid brown rice, as it is heavy and hard to digest. Favor white basmati rice, which is the least refined of all the white rices. You may have other white rices as well. Also try millet, buckwheat, oats, quinoa, and amaranth. If you are not gluten sensitive you may add non-GMO wheat (spelt, farro, kamut, and einkorn are some good types), barley, and rye.

Vegetables

You may have all the vegetables except those listed in the "Foods to Avoid" section above. The ancient doctors said that each vegetable has a problem associated with it—that it contains ingredients that are potentially bad for your health—but that cooking the vegetable would release the offending substance. As it turns out, they were right. For example, we now know that the cruciferous vegetables (such as broccoli, Brussels sprouts, cabbage, cauliflower, kale, and turnips) contain sulfur and are potential goitrogens, or foods that can disrupt thyroid function. We also know that the dark green leafy vegetables (such as chard, spinach, and kale) contain oxalic acid, which depletes the body of minerals, especially calcium and magnesium. However, cooking the vegetables releases or deactivates these harmful substances.

The majority of vegetables in your diet should be cooked anyway, as the chewing process alone isn't enough to break down the fibers, decreasing the amount of nutrients absorbed into the cells. Cooking vegetables softens the fibers, allowing for greater absorption. Better yet is to cook vegetables and coat them with ghee or olive oil. The fat, particularly in ghee, enhances absorption by carrying nutrients across the cell wall, which is composed of cholesterol.

You do not have to completely avoid raw vegetables, but they should comprise just a small percentage of the vegetables you eat during the week.

Fruits

All fruits are allowed, with the exception of bananas, which are somewhat channel clogging and can cause mucus and congestion to build up, especially if you have a head cold or lung infections. The smaller species of bananas sold in Asian markets are okay to consume.

Fruits digest and absorb quickly, so it is best to eat them by themselves, in between meals as a snack. Avoid raw fruits before the sun comes up, because your own digestive fire will not have ignited yet. For the same reason, avoid raw fruits once the sun has gone down, as your internal digestive fire goes to sleep now. Keep in mind that anything raw is always more difficult to digest so it's best to avoid raw fruits in the early and latter parts of the day.

Ayurveda recommends an apple or pear first thing in the morning as a way to encourage the timely removal of toxins and to boost ojas, or immunity. Since our digestive fire is low at this time, it is important to cook the fruit. Below is the recipe.

ॐ Cooked Apple or Pear

Peel and core the apple or pear, and cut it into quarters. Put the pieces in a small pot, and add enough water to cover them, along with 2 whole cloves (optional). Cook for a few minutes over medium-high heat, until the fruit is soft (different varieties of apples and pears will require different cooking times).

Fats and Oils

Vegetable Oils

Until recently it was thought that cholesterol clogged the arteries, so people were instructed to use vegetable oils instead of animal fats (like lard and butter), since they contain no cholesterol. However, these oils often contain large amounts of biologically active fats called omega-6 polyunsaturated fatty acids, which are extremely detrimental to our health. Polyunsaturated fatty acids tend to react with oxygen, which causes oxidation of the fat, leading to free radical formation and inflammation.

Because of this, many people are avoiding highly processed vegetable oils that are high in polyunsaturated omega-6s (canola oil, corn oil, safflower, sunflower, soybean oil, etc.) and returning to the use of oils with more monounsaturated fats—such as high-quality olive oil—and saturated fats—such as coconut oil and avocado oil. However, coconut and avocado oils are difficult to digest and are best avoided unless you have excellent digestion. A better alternative for a more saturated type of fat is ghee.

The ancient doctors, recognizing that butter is somewhat channel clogging, recommended clarifying the butter to make ghee, a process in which the dairy solids and water are removed, allowing the remaining fat easy entry into our cells. Ghee is nature's gift to us—it is a source of cholesterol that is easier to digest than any oil yet won't clog the arteries. I think if we knew more about ghee in this country it would receive its much deserved acclaim, as it is a form of cholesterol, which coconut and avocado oils are not, and the body has a great need for sources of cholesterol that are easy to digest yet won't clog the arteries.

The Health Benefits of Ghee

The Charaka Samhita, the foremost Ayurvedic text, states in sutra 27, verse 232, "out of all the oils fit for human consumption, ghee is the best to eat."

Ghee is rich in omega-3 fatty acids, which can help decrease levels of unhealthy cholesterol in the body. It is one of the best sources of butyric acid, which is, in turn, one of the most beneficial short-chain fatty acids. Butyric acid has been shown in recent research to decrease inflammation, particularly in the gastrointestinal tract. Butyric acid creates a fertile environment for beneficial bacteria to thrive, and it blocks the growth of bad bacteria in the gut. It also reduces leakage of undigested food particles through the intestinal walls (leaky gut) and repairs the gut's mucosal walls.

Ghee is 65 percent saturated fat, 25 percent monounsaturated fat, and 5 percent polyunsaturated fat. Its saturated fat content consists mainly of easily digested short-chain fatty acids. Short-chain fatty acids can be processed by the liver and burnt as energy, rather than passing into adipose tissue or contributing to weight gain.

In addition, ghee contains conjugated linoleic acid (CLA), which prevents inflammation in artery walls and hardening of the arteries (plaque formation). It increases the metabolic rate; enhances muscle growth and contributes to weight loss; lowers cholesterol and triglycerides; and lowers insulin resistance and thus prevents diabetes. It improves the ratio of lean mass to body fat; decreases fat deposition, especially in the abdomen; and prevents heart disease and cancer. Health food stores sell CLA to body builders; however, we do not recommend these synthetic sources, as they are known to cause side effects, such as upset stomach, nausea, diarrhea, fatigue, insulin resistance, and fatty liver. It turns out that ghee is one of the best natural sources of CLA.

The ancient doctors said that children who grew up eating ghee would be highly intelligent and women who ate ghee would be highly fertile. This was five thousand years ago before there were any microscopes! Now we know that both the brain and female hormones are made of cholesterol. This is also why ghee is described as the best food to improve memory and mental functions and at the same time to promote longevity.

Ghee imparts not only a beautiful glow to the skin but provides cholesterol so that the skin can convert sunlight into vitamin D. It is considered one of the best fats to nourish the fat tissue, which will in turn create healthy bones and lustrous hair.

Many bakeries, including those that supply health food stores, continue to use vegetable oils in their baked goods, thinking that they are a better alternative than butter. However, many of these oils have fairly low smoke points. The smoke or flash point occurs when the oil in the pan starts smoking, creating an acrid smell. The smoke is a sign of oxidation, which means that dangerous free radicals have formed. Ghee has one of the highest smoke points (485 degrees Fahrenheit) of any cooking oil; thus, ghee is recommended for use in baking and all high-temperature cooking.

You can purchase ready-made ghee, but make sure it comes from the butter of grass-fed cows. Ghee made from grain-fed cows does not confer the same health benefits. If you have the time and inclination, you can make your own ghee by following the two recipes below. The first is easy and takes less than a half hour to make, while the other is a two-day process.

You are probably asking yourself why you should make ghee that takes three days with all the trouble that it entails, when you could easily make it in one half hour? Good question!

The second and harder recipe requires you to make yogurt out of heavy cream, churn that into butter, and then make ghee out of that butter (rather than making ghee from premade butter). Culturing the cream was highly recommended in the ancient texts because it confers a higher level of prana than noncultured ghee. Also, the friendly bacteria in the yogurt cultures break the fats down into even smaller particles for better absorption. In addition, yogurt, having the qualities of fermentation (fire) lightens up the ghee, making it easier to digest. The element of fire is transformative and light in quality, and these qualities remain in the resultant ghee made from yogurt. In other words, the qualities of the yogurt have now been introduced into the butter.

An article published by K. S. Joshi in the *Journal of Ayurveda and Integrative Medicine* in 2014 demonstrated how the docosahexaenoic acid (DHA) content is significantly higher in ghee prepared by the traditional Ayurvedic method using cultured cream and concluded, "The findings suggest that ghee prepared by traditional Ayurvedic methods contains higher amounts of DHA and omega-3 long-chain polyunsaturated fatty acids, which are major components of retinal and brain tissues and remains important in the prevention of various diseases."

Cultured ghee is easier to digest for those suffering from lactose intolerance. Milk contains a natural sugar called lactose. In the body lactose has to be broken down into glucose and galactose, requiring an enzyme called lactase. Many people lack this enzyme, making it difficult to digest milk, hence the name "lactose intolerance." During the culturing of the milk the lactose is converted into lactic acid, making it more digestible for those lacking this enzyme.

Also, cultured ghee has twice the amount of conjugated linoleic acid than regular ghee, which builds more muscle and less fat, promoting weight loss.

As future studies are undertaken comparing the two types of ghee I am sure we will find more profound health benefits found in cultured ghee.

❧ Making Ghee: The Easy Recipe

For this recipe, all you need is unsalted grass-fed organic butter. Melt as much of the butter as you like (I usually work with a pound or 2 at a time) over low heat. Allow the butter to come to a very gentle simmer, but no more, or else you risk burning it. A white foam will form on top, and some solids will sink to the bottom. Occasionally skim off the white foam and discard it. After some time (about half an hour for 2 pounds of butter, a little less for 1 pound of butter and a little more for 3 pounds of butter), you will hear the butter crackling, and you will notice that you can see the bottom of the pot. The butter is now clarified. Skim the particles off the top again. Line a strainer with several layers of cheesecloth, set it over a glass bowl, and then pour the butter through the strainer. If the ghee in the bowl has any dairy solids remaining in it, strain it again.

Store ghee at room temperature. Due to its low moisture content and lack of dairy solids, it won't turn rancid at room temperature like butter and retains its freshness for about 1 month.

ॐ Making Ghee: The Harder Recipe

8 cups organic heavy cream

2 cups plain yogurt (preferably homemade)

1 1/2 teaspoons ProTren yogurt starter (see page 62)

Pour the cream into a pot. Bring to a boil, and then remove from the heat. Let cool to between 98 and 103 degrees Fahrenheit.

When the cream has cooled to the right temperature range, add the plain yogurt and yogurt starter, and whisk thoroughly. Cover the pot tightly, and place in the oven. Turn on the oven light. Let the mixture sit in the slightly warm oven for 8 to 10 hours. Then remove it from the oven, and refrigerate it for several hours, or overnight, until cold.

Add half of the yogurt cream to a food processor, and blend for about 5 minutes, or until curds of butter form. (Note: These curds will not form if the yogurt cream is warm; it must have been refrigerated for several hours for the fat to congeal.) Then add the other half of the yogurt cream, and also blend it until butter curds form.

Pour off the liquid (this is healthy buttermilk, or *takra*) through a strainer into a bowl. Now add about 1 cup of ice water to your food processor, and blend for about 1 minute. Again the buttermilk will separate out of the butter; pour that off through the strainer too.

Add another 1 cup of ice water to the butter in the food processor, blend for about another minute, and pour off that buttermilk.

Save the buttermilk, and store it in your refrigerator, where it will keep for about 3 days. This buttermilk has lots of friendly bacteria in it and makes a great probiotic; you can drink 1 cup a day at lunch, taking little sips between bites of food. You can also use it for baking.

Scrape the butter you just churned out of the food processor and into a bowl. Either squeeze the butter in your hands or twist it in a clean kitchen towel or butter muslin, extracting as much liquid as possible. (You might have to do this in two batches because you will have a lot of butter.)

Finally, put your butter in a pot, melt it over low heat, and let simmer very gently. Cook as instructed in the easy recipe above, skimming off any foam. You don't need to stir it. When the butter is crackling and clear enough that you can see through it to the bottom of the pot, remove it from the heat and pour it through several layers of cheesecloth into a glass bowl. If the ghee has any dairy solids remaining in it, strain it again, and the ghee should come out clear. Store at room temperature; it will stay fresh for about 1 month.

Olive Oil

Olive oil is a monounsaturated heart-healthy fat that we recommend. However, at least 80 percent of the oil sold in the United States does not meet the legal grade for extra-virgin olive oil. Journalist Tom Mueller, who has researched the industry, says that fraud runs rampant in the manufacturing and labeling. All too often bottlers dilute high-quality extra-virgin olive oil with lower-quality oils. Even worse, bottles labeled "extra-virgin olive oil" may not be olive oil at all but rather a seed oil, like sunflower, made to look and smell like olive oil with a few drops of chlorophyll and beta-carotene added.

The following brands failed to meet industry standards, according to published reports: Bertolli, Carapelli, Colavita, Filippo Berio, Mazola, Mezzetta, Newman's Own, Pompeian, Safeway, Star, and Whole Foods.

For certified olive oil, buy California Olive Ranch, Cobram Estate, Kirkland Organic, Lucero Ascolano, Lucini, and McEvoy Ranch Organic.

A good rule of thumb: If your olive oil turns solid when refrigerated, it's the real deal. If it remains liquid, it's been diluted with vegetable oils.

Olive oil is best used to "finish" a dish, as it can hydrogenate when heated. Some people recommend cooking with half ghee and half olive oil or adding some water to your olive oil when cooking with it to keep the temperature down.

Sesame Oil

Organic sesame oil is the only other oil we recommend for cooking. It can tolerate higher heat than olive oil. Of the three fats (sesame oil, olive oil, and ghee), ghee can handle the highest heat, and it is the easiest to digest.

Milk and Milk Products

Dairy is perhaps the most misunderstood of all the food groups. The ancient doctors said that every food you eat spends three to five days in each tissue before it progresses to the next. There are, as discussed earlier, seven tissues (blood plasma, blood, muscle, fat, bone, bone marrow, and reproductive fluids). This means that the food you eat today won't nourish the seventh tissue, the reproductive fluids, until about a month from now. The only exception to this rule is milk. It nourishes all seven tissues in one day! Thus milk is seen as one of the most nourishing foods of all. This is why babies can live exclusively off milk for the first year of life.

And yet, having seen thousands of patients over the last thirty years, I can attest to the fact that only once or twice a year will patients report to me that they include whole milk in their diet. Let's examine why that might be, looking at each of the common issues people have with milk.

I Get Congested When I Drink Milk

The ancient texts considered milk to be channel clogging and mucous producing if taken incorrectly, so they came up with strict prescriptions for its use.

- Always boil the milk to thin out the fat for better digestion and assimilation into the cells. In addition, boiling the milk will kill any infection in the milk, especially in the case of raw milk, but will not destroy the prana and the enzymes necessary to digest the milk in the same way that the industrial pasteurization of milk will. For pasteurized milk, you need only bring it to a boil and turn off the heat as it foams up. However, it is best to bring raw milk to a boil and let it simmer for a minute or two over a low heat to properly kill any potential pathogens in the milk.

- Never drink milk with fruits, vegetables, or proteins; consume it only with grains, dried fruits, nuts, and spices as it doesn't mix well in the stomach with other foods.
- Favor raw milk, which is easier to digest than processed milk.
- Favor nonhomogenized milk (look for a layer of cream on top) over homogenized milk.
- Drink whole milk, not low-fat or skim milk.
- Boil milk with cardamom pods, which help you digest the protein in the milk, and a piece of a cinnamon stick, which aids in the digestion of the carbohydrates in the milk.

Following these guidelines will prevent congestion from the ingestion of milk.

....

Why Nonhomogenized?

When milk is homogenized, its fat is broken down into smaller particles so that they will integrate throughout the milk, rather than separating out and rising to the top as cream. Homogenization is a standard treatment for most commercial milk.

However, the small fat globules that are formed during the homogenization process surround xanthine oxidase, a protein enzyme that is in cow's milk. Normally this enzyme would not survive the digestive process intact. But when milk is homogenized, the xanthine oxidase is absorbed intact into your bloodstream and eventually ends up in your heart, where it causes damage to the tissues and contributes to heart disease. This is why it is imperative to buy nonhomogenized whole milk, with the layer of cream at the top. You can shake the milk to disperse the fat before heating or cooking with it.

....

I'm Lactose Intolerant

My new patients often tell me that they avoid milk due to a dairy sensitivity, allergy, or intolerance. Usually they have been avoiding it for years, having switched over to almond or other nut milks, rice milk, soy milk, or goat's milk.

Most people are surprised to learn that by fixing their digestion and following the guidelines above to eliminate congestion caused by milk consumption, their sensitivity or allergy to milk will disappear.

If, however, you were born with a genetic lactose intolerance (which is far less common than the acquisition of a milk allergy due to disruption of the digestive system), you may have to exclude cow's milk from your diet. In this case, the ancient doctors said that goat's milk was the second most nourishing milk next to cow's milk. You might also try almond milk, but make your own. It will lose both prana and nutritional value as it sits on the shelf in the supermarket. Below is my recipe, which you can alter as you see fit. Add more almonds and less water if you like a thicker milk; use fewer almonds and more water for a thinner milk.

❧ Homemade Almond Milk

Soak ³/₄ cup of almonds with their skins on overnight in spring water. Rinse and then peel the almonds in the morning. Transfer them to a blender, and add enough water to cover them by about ³/₄ inch. Blend for 3 minutes. Strain through a nut milk bag. Drink immediately. You may sweeten the milk with a natural sweetener, such as raw honey, maple syrup, or organic cane sugar, if desired.

Other nut milks can be made in similar fashion. The processed rice milk on the market is less nourishing than the nut milks; avoid it. You should never consume soy milk, as soy depresses thyroid function.

A1 vs. A2 Milk

Cow's milk contains a type of protein, called beta-casein, that in recent years has been shown to exist in two forms, called A1 and

A2, which differ just slightly in the setup of their amino acid chains. Goat, sheep, water buffalo, and human breast milk all contain only A2-like beta-casein proteins. Cow's milk, however, varies. Some cows produce only A1, some only A2, and some have both proteins. In general, A1 is found in milk from Holsteins and other high-producing Western milk cows, while A2 predominates in Jersey, Guernsey, and most Asian and African breeds.

Both animal and human studies show that A2 milk is more easily digested than A1 milk. This is due to the fact that during the breakdown of A1 in the gut, a peptide fragment (a chain of amino acids) called BCM-7 is formed. This fragment slows digestion, causing inflammation and bloating, gas, abdominal pain, diarrhea, and constipation. This fragment is not formed with A2 milk.

As a result, many people who have been diagnosed as having "lactose intolerance" may actually simply be intolerant of A1 milk. Since most of the milk on the market today is a blend from many different cows, most of it contains a mix of A1 and A2 milk, and it will trigger digestive upset in almost anyone with an A1 sensitivity.

There are some limited sources of pure A2 milk around the country. If you can find it, it's worth trying, since milk is considered one of the most beneficial foods for our health. Many of our patients who thought they were lactose intolerant were surprised to find that they could digest A2 milk. As noted in the guidelines above, always boil whatever type of milk you can obtain, even A2 milk, to make it more digestible.

More research needs to be done to verify the health benefits of A2 milk, although the studies that have been reported in the literature so far show that it is easier to digest. One of the most exciting studies cited so far, published by R. Deth et al. in 2016, demonstrated that A2 milk promotes the production of the antioxidant glutathione in humans.

I Don't Want to Support the Dairy Industry Due to the Mishandling of Cows

The good news here is there are many small dairies that take good care of their cows, letting them roam in fields and eat grass. If you can find a small local dairy, you can inquire about their herd management practices.

In the early years of my Ayurvedic practice, I attended a lecture by Dr. Brihaspati Dev Triguna, a world-famous Ayurvedic physician known for his unique pulse diagnostic skills. He told us that it brings on bad karma to kill cows and eat their meat. In addition, when you do, you absorb the cow's stress hormones (adrenaline and cortisol), which were high at the time of slaughter. In contrast, he went on to say, the milk of the cow, which is given up in love for a calf, contains a loving, nurturing vibration, giving milk an added quality above and beyond other food sources.

Most patients tell me how nourished and calm they feel when sipping warm milk, and how well they sleep if they drink it before bed.

Milk Causes Autoimmune Diseases, Cancer, and Inflammation

If you drink poor-quality milk—highly processed, taken from grain-fed cows that are treated with antibiotics and hormones, pasteurized (heated to a high temperature for a long time, which kills the prana), and homogenized (making it even less bioavailable)—and you cannot digest the milk due to unaddressed digestive issues, then yes, the milk will turn into ama visha, a hot toxin, which can become the root of inflammatory conditions, autoimmune diseases, and cancer.

However, if you buy good-quality milk, correct your digestion, and drink the milk in the correct way (see page 179), then the milk becomes one of the most nourishing foods you can consume. And since it is soma producing and cooling, it actually helps lower inflammation and reduce the tendency toward autoimmune diseases and cancer.

I Don't Want the Fat, So I Only Drink Low-Fat Milk

We need fat to deliver calcium to our bones. The calcium in low-fat and skim milk products comes in one end of the digestive tract and out the other, never reaching the bones. Keep in mind that we now have an epidemic of osteopenia and osteoporosis in America, partly due to the use of low-fat milk products in concert with thyroid weakness.

If you want to decrease the fat content or heaviness of the milk, instead of drinking processed low-fat milk, dilute whole milk with water. This way you will avoid destroying the prana in the milk.

As you have now learned, most, if not all, thyroid conditions develop when vata is disturbed (from stress, rushing around, going to bed late, and so on). Warm milk is perhaps the best vata-pacifying food, with ghee being second, due to their heavy and unctuous nature. Therefore it is of utmost importance that you try to reincorporate milk into your diet.

Sweeteners

Many books have been written on the negative effects of refined white sugar on our health, describing its contribution to diabetes, tooth decay, obesity, heart disease, cancer, and poor cognitive functioning. Sugar is 50 percent glucose, which spikes our blood sugar, and 50 percent fructose, which goes straight to the liver, wreaking havoc there. Gary Taubes has written numerous articles in which he argues that sugar is not simply a source of excess calories, but a fundamental cause of obesity and type 2 diabetes. He emphasizes that "we must do more to discourage consumption while we improve our understanding of sugar's role."

Lisa Byrne describes the addictive qualities of sugar in her workbook, *Break the Sugar Habit:*

> Refined white sugar acts more like a drug than a food in our system . . . but it started as a whole plant. The sugar cane and beet plant in nature come complete with vitamins, minerals, fiber and phytochemicals like any other plant. And they have carbohydrates like any other plant in the form of sucrose. When sugar is refined they strip the sugarcane plant or beet plant of all its natural components, except the sucrose. The sucrose is concentrated into what we know as table sugar. When sucrose is part of the whole food it acts

like a food in your body, entering your system slowly, providing a range of nutrients in addition to energy. However, when the sucrose is isolated, it acts like a drug in your body, creating cycles of intense highs and lows in the blood sugar.

In fact, many people have withdrawal symptoms when they try to remove sugar from their diet.

In Ayurvedic terminology, we can say that the intelligence or prana in processed white sugar gets disturbed by the processing, and instead of nourishing our system, it will create side effects and toxicity, like any processed food.

There are numerous alternatives to processed white sugar. Some of these sweeteners should be avoided, while others are acceptable.

Sweeteners to Avoid

Agave nectar: Dr. Mishra never recommended agave nectar, as he felt it contained too much soma and was therefore heavy. Like many sweeteners found in their natural state, agave does contain some health benefits. And like most sugars, once it is processed and refined it is an unhealthy version far removed from its original state. When agave is processed into a syrup, fructose is formed. In fact, most agave nectars contain 70 to 90 percent fructose, more than what is found in high-fructose corn syrup. The high fructose in agave goes directly to the liver for further breakdown. Here it can build up fat deposits around the liver, contributing to nonalcoholic fatty liver disease. It also builds up triglycerides and creates insulin resistance, a risk factor for diabetes.

Artificial sweeteners: These are entirely synthetic and are toxic to the body. Aspartame, for example, is toxic to brain cells and is responsible for burning the myelin sheath, the covering of the nerve tissue, leading to multiple sclerosis and other demyelinating conditions.

High-fructose corn syrup: This sweetener ends up stored as fat in the liver and makes people resistant to leptin (a hormone), which increases appetite and contributes to weight gain.

Sucralose: Sucralose (Splenda) may derive from sucrose (sugar), but it is processed using chlorine and is another overly processed sugar that creates physiologic disturbance throughout the body.

Sugar alcohols: These sweeteners include xylitol, sorbitol, and erythritol and are made through a fermentation process of corn or sugar. Too much of these processed sweeteners can cause gastrointestinal distress: gas, bloating, and abdominal pain.

Sweeteners to Use

Blackstrap molasses: This sweetener is rich in iron, copper, manganese, selenium, vitamin B6, potassium, and calcium. In fact, just one tablespoon of blackstrap molasses provides more iron than a three-ounce serving of red meat. Molasses is the syrupy by-product of the process that turns sugarcane into refined white table sugar. Blackstrap molasses comes from the third boiling of raw cane sugar, concentrating its nutrients.

Brown rice syrup: This sweetener is extracted from brown rice that is fermented with enzymes to break down the starch. The liquid is then cooked down until it becomes a thick, amber-colored sweet syrup. If you are on a gluten-free diet, note that some brown rice syrups are fermented with barley enzymes. You can use this syrup as a substitute for corn syrup. It is fructose-free, so it has become a popular option among people with irritable bowel syndrome who experience intestinal distress when they consume fructose.

Coconut sugar: Coconut sugar is loaded with polyphenols, iron, zinc, calcium, potassium, antioxidants, phosphorus, and other phytonutrients. It is extracted from the sap of the blooms of the coconut palm, which is heated and evaporated to make coconut sugar. It serves as a suitable replacement for white sugar.

Date sugar: Date sugar is simply powdered dried dates, and it retains some of the nutrients found in whole dates, such as small amounts of fiber, calcium, potassium, and magnesium. It doesn't dissolve in drinks, so it is best sprinkled on foods. It is truly natural, since it hasn't been refined in any way, and contains fewer calories than table sugar.

Evaporated cane juice: This is a type of raw sugar made from fresh sugarcane juice that is evaporated and then crystallized. This sweetener is less refined than white sugar and therefore has more trace minerals and other nutrients found in sugarcane and causes less of a spike in blood sugar. It can be used as a substitute in recipes calling for sugar.

Maple syrup: Pure maple syrup, made from the boiled sap of maple trees, is packed with more minerals than honey. It also has high levels of antioxidants. Unlike honey, maple syrup is heat stable; you can cook with it. Just make sure that you are buying 100 percent pure maple syrup and not high-fructose corn syrup with "natural maple flavoring."

Natural brown sugar and raw sugar: These sugars retain some of the molasses from the evaporated sugarcane juice. Brown sugar can be up to 70 percent white sugar with varying amounts of molasses; the amount of molasses depends on how much was spun out when the sugar crystals were centrifuged.

Turbinado, demerara, and so-called "raw" sugars are spun in a centrifuge long enough to remove almost all of the molasses.

Muscovado, panela, piloncillo, chancaca, jaggery, and other natural dark brown sugars have been minimally centrifuged or not at all. These sugars are usually made in smaller factories in developing nations, where they are produced with traditional practices that do not make use of industrialized vacuum evaporators or centrifuges. They are usually boiled in open pans on wood-fired stoves until the sugarcane juice reaches the crystallizing point. They are then poured into molds to solidify or into cooling pans where they are worked vigorously to produce a granulated brown sugar that retains more molasses and therefore more nutrients than the more highly processed brown sugars on the market.

Raw honey: Minimally processed raw honey has a low glycemic index, which means it won't create the spikes and valleys in blood sugar levels that white sugar does—it is slowly absorbed into the bloodstream. It contains numerous antioxidants, enzymes, iron, zinc, potassium, calcium, phosphorus, vitamin B₆, riboflavin, and niacin, and it is highly beneficial to your health. Research shows that it has antimicrobial properties effective for fighting cold symptoms. (Pasteurized honey, on the other hand, has no health benefits.)

Ayurveda considers all sweeteners to be cooling except for honey, which is heating. Honey is therefore helpful when you have a cold or need to burn ama out of the channels. This is why people sip hot tea with honey when they are sick (the sweet taste of other sweeteners would simply create more kapha, increasing congestion). Make sure, however, to add honey to the tea only once it has cooled to the point that you can sip it without burning yourself. Heat denatures honey, forming compounds that contribute to ill health. Do not use honey in baking—just drizzle on top of food for best results.

Stevia: Stevia sweetener is extracted from the leaves of the stevia plant. It contains zero calories and is one of the more natural sweeteners. While it is not a significant source of nutrition, the best thing about stevia is that it will not affect blood sugar levels, making it a great sugar alternative for diabetics. It is also calorie-free. However, be wary of Truvia; this commercial sweetener is made in part from stevia extract, along with a sugar alcohol, and contains some genetically engineered ingredients.

Sucanat: Sucanat is made by extracting the juice from freshly cut sugarcane, then heating and drying it. It is just as sweet as table sugar but has a stronger molasses flavor. It retains the nutrients found in the sugarcane juice, unlike processed table sugar and turbinado sugar.

Nuts and Seeds

According to Ayurveda, nuts and seeds contain heat. As a result, we recommend that you soak nuts and seeds in spring water overnight to cool them down. As they absorb the water, they soften, which allows for better digestion and cell absorption.

Nuts and Seeds to Avoid

Chia, hemp, and pumpkin seeds: Avoid these seeds, which are considered channel clogging.

Flax: Flaxseeds and flaxseed oil are considered too heating to the liver and spleen and are never recommended in the diet.

Peanuts: Peanuts are not recommended because they contain a mold that produces aflatoxin. Aflatoxin is a known carcinogen associated with liver cancer. It has also been shown to stunt growth in children.

Prescriptions for Nuts and Seeds

All the other nuts and seeds are recommended with these simple caveats:

- Peel the skin off almonds after soaking them overnight, as the skin is indigestible.
- Lightly toast sesame seeds and then grind them for better digestion and absorption.
- Don't overconsume cashews, which are heavy in nature.
- Don't eat more than a handful or two of nuts and seeds at a time, as they are somewhat heavy and hard to digest.
- Refrain from nut butters, which are hard to digest and clog the channels. Freshly made nut milks are much lighter and easier to digest and are therefore more nourishing than the nut butters.

All nuts and seeds are good sources of dietary fiber and are highly nourishing. They provide B vitamins, including folate; vitamin E; minerals, including calcium, iron, zinc, potassium, and magnesium; antioxidant minerals, including selenium, manganese, and copper; and other phytochemicals, such as antioxidant compounds (flavonoids and resveratrol) and plant sterols. They provide large quantities of healthy monounsaturated and polyunsaturated fats and moderate amounts of protein.

Since they are hard to digest, it is recommended that children in their first two years of life avoid nuts in their diets.

DAILY ROUTINE (DINACHARYA)

Dinacharya is the Sanskrit word for daily routine: *din* means "day" and *charya* means "to follow." Dinacharya is a concept in Ayurvedic medicine that considers the cycles of nature and bases our daily activities around these cycles. If we attune our bodies to the fundamental laws of nature, Ayurveda tells us, we can attain optimal health.

To understand these concepts, we begin our discussion with the vata, pitta, and kapha times of the day:

- Kapha periods: 6 a.m. to 10 a.m. and 6 p.m. to 10 p.m.
- Pitta periods: 10 a.m. to 2 p.m. and 10 p.m. to 2 a.m.
- Vata periods: 2 a.m. to 6 a.m. and 2 p.m. to 6 p.m.

This means that the elements of vata, pitta, and kapha are predominant during these hours. You can use this information as a basic blueprint to map out your day's activities, and by doing so, you will keep these elements of vata, pitta, and kapha balanced in your physiology.

The body craves routine, and it is much easier to stay healthy if you wake up at roughly the same time every day, eat your meals at the same time, and go to bed at the same time. If you are haphazard in your schedule, vata will get thrown out of balance. Vata is considered the "leading dosha," meaning that once it is disrupted, the other two doshas, pitta and kapha, will slowly imbalance as well.

A good example is if you go to bed late or at varying times, skip breakfast, eat on the run, and eat at varying times of the day and night as you rush through the day with an ever-changing schedule. Now vata is disturbed. Next, you might notice that your digestion isn't optimal— you may start belching or having more gas as pitta gets disturbed. Finally, you'll start putting on weight as the body dumps the undigested food into your abdomen or upper thighs as kapha now becomes disrupted.

Let's now look at a synchronized day, according to the vata, pitta, and kapha times of day.

Vata Time: 2 a.m. to 6 a.m.

This is the time of day when vata becomes active in the physiology. It is best to wake up before the sun rises. The hour of sunrise is different at different times of the year, but roughly 6 a.m. is considered an optimal time for rising. Try to train your body to have a bowel movement first thing in the morning to rid your body of the previous day's wastes.

This is also the time of day for meditation, prayer, or spiritual practice. The ancient doctors said that an hour and a half before sunrise was considered the *brahma muhurta,* or "time of Brahma." During this time of the day, soma, agni, and marut are perfectly balanced, so waking up during this time is conducive to producing a balanced, serene mind. One of the foundational Ayurvedic texts, the Astanga Hrdayam, states that "a healthy person should get up (from bed) during brahma muhurta, to protect his life" (Astanga Hrdayam, vol. 1, 2:1). It is also considered an ideal time for study and to obtain *brahma* (knowledge). The ancients went so far as to say that it is also the best time to conceive a child—the vibrations in the environment and your body are most settled and blissful, which can produce a well-rounded, happy baby.

Kapha Time: 6 a.m. to 10 a.m.

This is the time of day when kapha is more active both in the environment and in our bodies. Since kapha is considered slow, dense, and somewhat heavy, if you sleep during this time (unless you are sick and confined to bed, which is allowed), you will feel a sense of lethargy and depression for the rest of the day. So again, it is best to arise before 6 a.m. This is the best time of day to exercise to dispel the heaviness from your body. Yoga, stretching, walking, and various other forms of exercise are recommended regularly to help promote relaxation, digestion, elimination, and sound sleep. This is the time to bathe as well.

Your internal agni, or digestive fire, is slowly awakening now, which is why you don't usually feel strong hunger upon awakening. Then as the sun comes up, your agni will rise as well and you become ready to eat. We recommend warm cooked food for breakfast, as opposed to cold food, which will put out the digestive fire as it is trying to ignite. Try stewed fruit, followed by cooked grains (with milk, if you can digest it) and cooked eggs. Avoid yogurt and smoothies.

Pitta Time: 10 a.m. to 2 p.m.

When the sun is highest in the sky, your internal agni is the most active as well. This is the time of day to eat your heaviest meal, since digestion is strongest now. Conversely, this is the worst meal to skip (although it is not recommended that you skip any meal), as the strong digestive fire is looking for food to digest. If there is no food, this internal heat can spread into the body, creating inflammation, headaches, irritability (think how children become when they are overly hungry and you forgot to bring their snacks!), rashes, and other pitta-aggravated conditions. This can be the underlying cause of high blood pressure, as the hot blood pounds against the arterial walls. I have resolved many cases of headaches and high blood pressure just by telling patients to always eat on time and never skip or delay a meal.

Vata Time: 2 p.m. to 6 p.m.

This time of day is good for study and work, since vata, which stimulates mental activity, predominates now.

Kapha Time: 6 p.m. to 10 p.m.

It is best to eat a light dinner, since the digestive fire is now on its way out. The slow, dull energy of kapha starts to again take over as we now prepare our bodies to unwind for sleep. It is best to avoid stimulating activities such as long telephone conversations, work, or computer or cell phone use; instead, try walking in the moonlight or reading a good book to allow sleep to overcome you.

Pitta Time: 10 p.m. to 2 a.m.

During the preceding kapha time period, it is of utmost importance that you go to bed at the first impulse of drowsiness. Resist the temptation to stay up; if you do, you will enter pitta time and get a second wind. What you are in fact doing is calling on the endocrine system to kick in to produce more adrenaline and cortisol. Now you will be able to stay up, but you unknowingly pushed your body out of balance. As the adrenaline circulates in your bloodstream, it will become difficult to sink into a blissful, uninterrupted, rejuvenating sleep. This is one of the basic causes of thyroid (and other endocrine) problems.

REMEMBER JUDY?

I no longer have to keep tissues close by when Judy comes for her biannual exam. Supple and energetic, she's lost weight and is the envy of her yoga class. Many of her friends ask her for advice on how to get in better shape. She no longer suffers anxiety listening to her heart rhythms at night because they are normal. Her hair is full and lustrous. And the best part is, she accomplished all this without having to resort to using pharmaceuticals or nutraceuticals.

CONCLUSION
Visionary Medicine

A few years ago Siddartha Mukherjee, a cancer researcher and Pulitzer Prize–winning author, took the stage for a TED talk and offered a tantalizing vision pointing to a new model of medicine. He mused about the possibility of using stem cells to make new bone and cartilage, a development that would revolutionize the treatment of arthritis. He suggested that the day may come when we can create organs outside the body for implantation.

His medical evangelism was well placed. On the horizon are a number of inspiring and life-changing technologies. Imagine diabetics being able to measure their blood glucose levels from tears. Picture a literal cutting-edge development where an intelligent surgical knife uses electrical current to heat tissue and make incisions without blood loss. Envision advances in radiology that show the percentage of your cells that are cancer-free. Contemplate a wearable sensor that can report a stroke in real time to medical professionals and call an ambulance for an incapacitated patient.

It is clear that we are on the precipice of astonishing advances in medicine. However, as I have argued in this book, nothing can replace the wisdom passed down through the ages. Remember, Ayurveda is built on foundational principles. It is the original healing system, based on pure knowledge that remains unwavering no matter the era.

What can and must change is the interaction between Ayurvedic physicians (or any holistic practitioners, for that matter) and the medical establishment. In my vision of the future, there is a place for collaboration and open-minded inquiry—always in the name of helping patients regain their health.

Doctors of the future will finally bow to the stampede of patients seeking holistic care and recognize the value of Ayurveda and how it fills gaps in modern medicine. They will know just enough about Ayurveda to feel comfortable referring patients to us and, more important, when a referral is necessary. They will consider us members of the health care team who are capable of addressing conditions before they become difficult to treat and manage. They will acknowledge that a systemic approach that goes beyond pharmaceuticals may be necessary and beneficial in many instances.

Doctors of the future will also listen to their patients, who know their bodies better than anyone. They will not dismiss patients who present with numerous symptoms despite "normal" blood work and diagnostic tests. What a boon it would be for patients to no longer have to leave their doctor's office feeling like hypochondriacs in need of antidepressants just because, seemingly, nothing is wrong.

As fanciful as my vision sounds, it is quite practical. In my ideal world, a model based on early intervention, when feasible, will alleviate some of the pressures on our health care system. More emphasis on prevention in the form of good diet, good daily routine, and effective cleansing techniques could relieve doctors of the crushing burden of treating so many seriously ill patients whose problems were allowed to fester.

Yes, we should continue to explore the frontiers of medicine. There are many lifesaving procedures and methodologies to come. But just think about a world in which we reduce the number of costly surgeries, the use of high-priced pharmaceuticals, and the frequency of doctor visits.

This is the real answer to our crisis in health care—patients who are so healthy that they don't much require the conventional medical system, which would save billions of dollars and make it possible for everyone to have health insurance.

On that hopeful note, let me close the way I began, with a case history, this one circa 2080:

After a stressful year acclimating to her new job as a high-powered CEO in Manhattan, Susan noticed that she wasn't feeling her usual self.

She was sluggish and had put on an extra twenty pounds, even though she hadn't changed her diet in any way. She also noticed more hair falling out and was feeling rather depressed, even though she had her son's wedding in a few months to look forward to.

She turned to her holographic keyboard to access information about her physiology. When she did, Susan found that nothing seemed awry; all values were normal. Using her super smart phone, she could see a 3D image of the cells in her body, and she quickly found the culprit—her thyroid gland's cells were malfunctioning.

Her doctor immediately downloaded this image onto his own super smart phone and told her to come in for a consultation. He gave her three options: One was to implant tiny microchips into her thyroid gland, using her own stem cells to create new thyroid cells.

The second was to use light to control the cells in her thyroid gland. Specifically, Susan would genetically modify her neurons with light-sensitive ion channels and at least theoretically rehabilitate and normalize her thyroid cells.

His third option was to consult with the Ayurvedic doctor who was part of his diverse practice of endocrinologists, holistic practitioners, and bodyworkers.

Both she and her doctor decided to start with the Ayurvedic approach, which was the least invasive, since she could always resort to the other methods if this treatment failed.

Following her examination, the Ayurvedic doctor recommended a treatment plan that took a whole-body approach to fixing the thyroid. She would go to bed early, cook healthy food at home, and take herbs to support her thyroid and improve her gallbladder function.

In no time, Susan began to perk up with newfound energy. She lost weight easily, and her thyroid cells began to function normally again. Her endocrinologist, the Ayurvedic physician, and, of course, Susan couldn't have been happier.

To all the Susans who are suffering needlessly, you don't have to wait for 2080 or the next century. The medicine of the future is here now. All we need is the foresight to take advantage of it.

Resources

Banyan Botanicals
800-953-6424 or 541-488-9525 (if calling from outside the USA)
www.banyanbotanicals.com
Certified organic, sustainably sourced, and fairly traded herbs, Ayurvedic tablets, liquid extracts, oils and balms, soaps, and skin-care products

Bhagavat Life
www.bvtlife.com
Ayurvedic cooking classes and professional culinary training teaching all aspects of the diet recommended in this book

Bliss Alchemy
www.blissalchemy.net
Offering body creams, facial cleansers, organic cultured ghee, organic jams, masalas, flower essences, online courses, Ayurvedic workshops, postpartum workshops, cooking classes, and other body and facial therapies

Chandi, LLC
www.chandika.com
888-324-2634 (toll-free in the USA) or 818-709-1005 (if calling from outside the USA)
Over seven hundred high-quality Ayurvedic remedies, personal-care products, spices, cultured ghee, magnesium chloride products, and more, all developed by award-winning herbal formulator Vaidya Rama Kant Mishra. These include soma salt, transdermal magnesium, vitamin D, glutathione, and various herbal transdermal creams and herbal glyceride drops (in which the vibration of the herb is captured in an organic yellow squash syrup) to be used when the patient's liver is too hot for the ingestion of crude physical herbal tablets or teas.

Divya's Kitchen
divyaskitchen.com
25 First Avenue, New York, NY 10003
212-477-4834
Flavorful and inventive Ayurvedic cooking based on the dietary guidelines recommended in this book

Frontier Co-op
www.frontiercoop.com
844-550-6200
A member-owned cooperative supporting natural living since 1976, providing highest-quality organic, fair-trade bulk herbs, teas, foods, and spices

Gita Nagari Eco Farm and Sanctuary
https://gnecofarm.org
534 Gita Nagari Road, Port Royal, PA 17082
717-527-4101
A nonprofit organization established in 1974, Gita Nagari is home to the first and only certified slaughter-free dairy farm in North America, based on the ancient principle of *ahimsa,* or nonviolence. A good source of A2 milk, yogurt, and freshly made curd cheeses.

Maharishi Ayurveda Products
www.mapi.com
800-255-8332 or 641-469-6940 (if calling from outside the USA)
Suppliers of Ayurvedic herbal supplements, skin-care and antiaging products, massage oils, teas, food, and spices

Miller's Organic Farm
www.millersorganicfarm.com
648 Mill Creek School Road, Bird in Hand, PA 17505
717-556-0672
A source of A2 raw milk, which can be shipped overnight on ice anywhere in the mainland United States

Mountain Rose Herbs
www.mountainroseherbs.com
P.O. Box 50220, Eugene, OR 97405
800-879-3337 (inside the USA) or 541-741-7307 (if calling from outside the USA)
An extensive selection of certified organic, fair-trade spices, herbs, teas, and botanical products

ProTren Intelligent Probiotics
www.protren.com
888-381-1887
Protren specializes in manufacturing the highest pharmaceutical grade quality probiotic supplements, setting a global standard of excellence. ProTren is committed to supporting health care practitioners and their patients through education, accessibility, quality and designated expert sales consultants. Probiotic cultures are 100% potency guaranteed.

Pure Indian Foods
www.pureindianfoods.com
Top-quality supplements and products in health, beauty, and fitness, including organic yellow split mung dal, chana dal, flours, cultured ghee, and more

Radiance Dairy
1745 Brookville Road, Fairfield, Iowa 52556
641-919-8554
Radiance Dairy is an organic, pasture-based dairy farm located in Fairfield, Iowa, supplying organic, sustainable, grass-fed A2 milk.

Starwest Botanicals
www.starwest-botanicals.com
800-800-4372
The premier site for bulk and wholesale herbs, spices, teas, herbal capsules, and more

SV Ayurveda
svayurveda.com
A website containing various forms of e-courses, a blog, and a newsletter giving information based on the teachings of Vaidya Rama Kant Mishra

Udder Milk Creamery Co-op
uddermilk.com
201-428-8745 or 973-413-9585
A source of A2 raw milk and 100 percent grass-fed dairy products and meats, health and beauty products, honey, grains, healthy snacks, preserves, jams and sauces, pet food, and more

References

PREFACE

Chaudhary, A., and N. Singh. "Contribution of World Health Organization in the Global Acceptance of Ayurveda." *Journal of Ayurveda and Integrative Medicine* 2 (2011): Oct–Dec, 179–86.

1. WHAT IS AYURVEDA?

Frawley, David. *Ayurvedic Healing.* Twin Lakes, Wisc.: Lotus Press, 2000.

Lad, Vasant. *Ayurveda: The Science of Self-Healing.* Santa Fe, N.Mex.: Lotus Press, 1984.

Mishra, Rama Kant. *SVA Pulse and Marma Course Manual.* Los Angeles: Adishakti, 2014.

Morrison, Judith H. *The Book of Ayurveda: A Holistic Approach to Health and Longevity.* London: Gaia Books, 1995.

Verma, Vinod. *Ayurveda: A Way of Life.* York Beach, Maine: Samuel Weiser, 1995.

2. THE THYROID GLAND AND ENDOCRINE SYSTEM

Abdulkhaliq, M., et al. "Effects of Lactobacillus acidophilus on Pituitary-Thyroid Axis in Growing Rat." *Advances in Animal and Veterinary Sciences* 3 (2015): 269–76.

Adler, S. M., et al. "The Nonthyroidal Illness Syndrome." *Endocrinology and Metabolism Clinics of North America* 36 (2007): 657–72.

Albright, F. "The Effect of Vitamin D on Calcium and Phosphorus Metabolism: Studies on Four Patients." *Journal of Clinical Investigation* 17 (1938): 305–15.

Asprey, D. "The Benefits of Vitamin D—Why It's the Sexiest Vitamin Around." Blog post on Dr. Sarah Gottfried, MD, April 8, 2014. www.saragottfriedmd .com/the-benefits-of-vitamin-d-why-its-the-sexiest-vitamin-around.

Baeke, F., et al. "Vitamin D: Modulator of the Immune System." *Current Opinion in Pharmacology* 10 (2010): 482–96.

Barnes, Broda O. *Hypothyroidism*. New York: HarperCollins, 1976.

Belenchia, A. M., et al. "Correcting Vitamin D Insufficiency Improves Insulin Sensitivity in Obese Adolescents." *American Journal of Clinical Nutrition* 97 (2013): 774–81.

Bertone-Jonson, E. R. "Vitamin D and the Occurrence of Depression: Causal Association or Circumstantial Evidence?" *Nutrition Reviews* 67 (2009): 481–92.

Bowthorpe, Janie A. *Stop the Thyroid Madness*. 2nd ed. Fredericksburg, Tex.: Laughing Grape, 2014.

Caldwell, G., et al. "A New Strategy for Thyroid Function Testing," *Lancet* 325 (1985): 1117–19.

Cantorna, M. T., et al. "Vitamin D Status, 1,25-dihydroxyvitamin D3, and the Immune System." *American Journal of Clinical Nutrition* 80 (2004): 171S–720S.

Carter, J. N., et al. "Effect of Severe, Chronic Illness on Thyroid Function." *Lancet* 2, no. 7887 (1974): 971–74.

Chopra, I. J., et al. "Thyroid Function in Nonthyroidal Illnesses." *Annals of Internal Medicine* 98, no. 6 (1983): 946–57.

Cui, X., et al. "The Vitamin D Receptor in Dopamine Neurons; Its Presence in Human Substantia Nigra and Its Ontogenesis in Rat Midbrain." *Neuroscience* 236 (2013): 77–87.

Ebert, E. C. "The Thyroid and the Gut." *Journal of Clinical Gastroenterology* 44 (2010): 402–6.

Edlund, C., and C. E. Nord. "Effect on the Human Normal Microflora of Oral Antibiotics for Treatment of Urinary Tract Infections." *Journal of Antimicrobial Chemotherapy* 46 (2000): 41–48.

Fatourechi, V. "Subclinical Thyroid Disease." *Mayo Clinic Proceedings* 4 (2001): 413–17.

Finegold, S. M., et al. "Comparative Effects of Broad Spectrum Antibiotics on Non-Spore-Forming Anaerobes and Normal Bowel Flora." *Annals New York Academy of Sciences* 145 (1967): 269–81.

Friesema, E. C. H., et al. "Thyroid Hormone Transporters." *Biochemical Society Transactions: Transporters 2004: International Symposium on Membrane Transport and Transporter* 33 (2005): 228–32.

Goswami, R., et al. "Prevalence of Vitamin D Deficiency and Its Relationship with Thyroid Autoimmunity in Asian Indians: A Community-Based Survey." *British Journal of Nutrition* 102 (2009): 382–86.

Greenblatt, J. M. "Psychological Consequences of Vitamin D Deficiency." Blog post on the Psychology Today, November 14, 2011. www.psychologytoday.com/us/blog/the-breakthrough-depression-solution/201111/psychological-consequences-vitamin-d-deficiency.

Groves, N. J., et al. "Adult Vitamin D Deficiency Leads to Behavioural and Brain Neurochemical Alterations in C57BL/6J and BALB/c Mice." *Behavioural Brain Research* 241 (2013): 120–31.

Hanker, J. P. "Gastrointestinal Disease and Oral Contraception." *American Journal of Obstetrics and Gynecology* 163 (1990): 2204–7.

Harris, A. R. C., et al. "Effect of Starvation, Nutriment Replacement, and Hypothyroidism on In Vitro Hepatic T4 to T3 Conversion in the Rat." *Metabolism* 27 (1978): 1680–90.

Hodgson, H., et al. "The Relationship between the Thyroid Gland and the Liver." *Quarterly Journal of Medicine* 95 (2002): 559–69.

Holick, M. F. "Sunlight and Vitamin D for Bone Health and Prevention of Autoimmune Diseases, Cancers, and Cardiovascular Disease." *American Journal of Clinical Nutrition* 80 (2004): 1678S–88S.

Holick, M. F. "Vitamin D Deficiency." *New England Journal of Medicine* 3357 (2007): 266–81.

Holick, M. F., et al. "Vitamin D and Skin Physiology: A D-Lightful Story." *Journal of Bone and Mineral Research* 22 (2007): V28–33.

Holtorf, K. "Thyroid Hormone Transport into Cellular Tissue." *Journal of Restorative Medicine* 3 (2014): 53–68.

Huang, M., and Y. Liaw. "Clinical Associations between Thyroid and Liver Diseases." *Journal of Gastroenterology and Hepatology* 10 (1995): 344–50.

Ingarbar, S. H., and L. E. Braverman. "Active Form of the Thyroid Hormone." *Annual Review of Medicine* 26 (1975): 443–49.

Kamen, D. L., et al. "Vitamin D and Molecular Actions on the Immune System: Modulation of Innate and Autoimmunity." *Journal of Molecular Medicine* 88 (2010): 441–50.

Kesby, J. P., et al. "Developmental Vitamin D Deficiency Alters Dopamine-Mediated Behaviors and Dopamine Transporter Function in Adult Female Rats." *Psychopharmacology* 208 (2010): 159–68.

Khalili, H., et al. "Hormone Therapy Increases Risk of Ulcerative Colitis but Not Crohn's Disease." *Gastroenterology* 143 (2012): 1199–206.

Khalili, H. et al. "Oral Contraceptives, Reproductive Factors and Risk of Inflammatory Bowel Disease." *Gut* 62 (2013): 1153–59.

Kharrazian, Datis. *Why Do I Still Have Thyroid Symptoms?* Carlsbad, Calif.: Elephant Printing, 2010.

Kilon, F. M., et al. "The Effect of Altered Thyroid Function on the Ultrastructure of the Human Liver." *American Journal of Medicine* 50 (1971): 317–24.

Kim, S., et al. "Relationship between Serum Vitamin D Levels and Symptoms of Depression in Stroke Patients." *Annals of Rehabilitative Medicine* 40 (2016): 120–25.

Kivity, S., et al. "Vitamin D and Autoimmune Thyroid Diseases." *Cellular & Molecular Immunology* 8 (2011): 243–48.

Klee, G. G., et al. "Biochemical Testing of Thyroid Function." *Endocrinology and Metabolism Clinics of North America* 26 (1997): 763–75.

Koulouri, O., et al. "Pitfalls in the Measurement and Interpretation of Thyroid Function Tests." *Best Practice & Research: Clinical Endocrinology & Metabolism* 27 (2013): 745–62.

Kunc, M., et al. "Microbiome Impact on Metabolism and Function of Sex, Thyroid, Growth and Parathyroid Hormones." *Acta Biochimica Polonica* 63, no. 2 (2016): 189–201.

Larsen, P. R., et al. "Relationships between Circulating and Intracellular Thyroid Hormones: Physiological and Clinical Implications." *Endocrine Reviews* 2 (1981): 87–102.

Madden, J. A. J., et al. "Effect of Probiotics on Preventing Disruption of the Intestinal Microflora Following Antibiotic Therapy." *International Immunopharmacology* 5 (2005): 1091–97.

Martin, I. S., et al. "Subclinical Thyroid Disease: Scientific Review and Guidelines for Diagnosis and Management," *Journal of the American Medical Association* 291, no. 2 (2004): 228–38.

McDermott, M. T., et al. "Subclinical Hypothyroidism Is Mild Thyroid Failure and Should Be Treated." *Journal of Clinical Endocrinology & Metabolism* 86 (2001): 4585–90.

McGregor, B. "Extra-Thyroidal Factors Impacting Thyroid Hormone Homeostasis." *Journal of Restorative Medicine* 4 (2015): 40–49.

Mora, J. R., et al. "Vitamin Effects on the Immune System: Vitamins A and D Take Centre Stage." *Nature Reviews: Immunology* 8 (2008): 685–98.

Myers, S. P. "The Causes of Intestinal Dysbiosis." *Alternative Medicine Review* 9 (2004): 180–97.

Nicolaysen, R. "Studies upon the Mode of Action of Vitamin D: The Influence of Vitamin D on the Absorption of Calcium and Phosphorus in the Rat." *Biochemistry Journal* 31 (1937): 122–29.

Patil, A. D. "Link between Hypothyroidism and Small Intestinal Bacterial Overgrowth." *Indian Journal of Endocrinological Metabolism* 18 (2014): 307–9.

Patrick, R. P., et al. "Vitamin D and the Omega-3 Fatty Acids Control Serotonin Synthesis and Action, Part 2: Relevance for ADHD, Bipolar Disorder, Schizophrenia, and Impulsive Behavior." *Federation of American Societies for Experimental Biology* 29 (2015): 2207–22.

Piudowski, P., et al. "Vitamin D Effects on Musculoskeletal Health, Immunity, Autoimmunity, Cardiovascular Disease, Dementia and Mortality." *Autoimmunity Reviews* 12 (2013): 976–89.

Ringel, M. D., and E. L. Mazzaferri. "Subclinical Thyroid Dysfunction—Can There Be a Consensus about the Consensus?" *Journal of Clinical Endocrinology & Metabolism* 90 (2005): 588–90.

Shafer, R. B., et al. "Gastrointestinal Transit in Thyroid Disease." *Gastroenterology* 86 (1984): 852–55.

Shimada, T., et al. "FGF-23 Is a Potent Regulator of Vitamin D Metabolism and Phosphate Homeostasis." *Journal of Bone and Mineral Research* 19 (2004): 429–35.

Simpson, S. J., et al. "Nutritional Impacts on Immunity, Microbiome and Metabolic Health: Lessons from Insects." *Australasian Medical Journal* 6 (2013): 580–685.

Smuts, Jan Christiaan. *Holism and Evolution.* Whitefish, Mont.: Kessinger Publishing, 1927.

Tompkins, Peter, and Christopher Bird. *The Secret Life of Plants.* New York: Harper & Row, 1989.

Trinko, J. R., et al. "Vitamin D3: A Role in Dopamine Circuit Regulation, Diet-Induced Obesity and Drug Consumption." *eNeuro* 3, no. 2 (2016): ii.

Van der Waaij, D., et al. "Colonization Resistance of the Digestive Tract in Conventional and Antibiotic-Treated Mice." *Epidemiology & Infection* 69 (1971): 405–11.

Williams, D. "Detox Naturally with Cilantro and Clay." Dr. David Williams, www.drdavidwilliams.com/cilantro-clay-for-detoxification.

Zhongjion, X., et al. "Lack of Vitamin D Receptor Is Associated with Reduced Epidermal Differentiation and Hair Growth." *Journal of Investigative Dermatology* 118 (2002): 11–16.

3. THE ROOT CAUSES OF THYROID MALFUNCTION

Abascal, K., and E. Yarnell. "Cilantro—Culinary Herb or Miracle Medicinal Plant?" *Alternative and Complementary Therapies* 18, Published Online: October 12, 2012. https://doi.org/10.1089/act.2012.18507.

Agmon-Levin, N., et al. "Vitamin D in Systemic and Organ-Specific Autoimmune Diseases." *Clinical Reviews in Allergy & Immunology* 45 (2013): 256–66.

Albert, B. B., et al. "Supplementation with a Blend of Krill and Salmon Oil Is Associated with Increased Metabolic Risk in Overweight Men." *American Journal of Clinical Nutrition* 102, no. 1 (2015): 49–57.

Allred, C. D., et al. "Soy Diets Containing Varying Amounts of Genistein (isoflavone) Stimulate Growth of Estrogen-Dependent Tumors in a Dose-Dependent Manner." *Cancer Research* 61 (2001): 5045–50.

Andreeva, V. A., et al. "B Vitamin and/or Omega-3 Fatty Acid Supplementation and Cancer: Ancillary Findings from the Supplementation with Folate, Vitamins B6 and B12, and/or Omega-3 Fatty Acids Randomized Trial." *Archives of Internal Medicine* 172 (2012): 540–47.

Appleby, P. N., et al. "The Oxford Vegetarian Study: An Overview." *American Journal of Clinical Nutrition* 70 (1999): 525s–31s.

Arit, W., et al. "Adrenal Insufficiency." *Lancet* 361 (2003): 1881–93.

Armario, A., et al. "Effect of Acute and Chronic Psychogenic Stress on

Corticoadrenal and Pituitary-Thyroid Hormones in Male Rats." *Hormone Research in Paediatrics* 20 (1984): 241–45.

Armstrong, B. K., et al. "Diet and Reproductive Hormones: A Study of Vegetarian and Nonvegetarian Postmenopausal Women." *Journal of the National Cancer Institute* 67 (1981): 761–67.

Arthur, J. R., et al. "Selenium Deficiency, Thyroid Hormone Metabolism and Thyroid Hormone Deiodinases." *American Journal of Clinical Nutrition* 57 (1993): 236S–39S.

Astwood, E. B. "The Chemical Nature of Compounds Which Inhibit the Function of the Thyroid Gland." *Journal of Pharmacology and Experimental Therapeutics* 78 (1943): 79–89.

Azizi, F., et al. "Effect of Dietary Composition on Fasting-Induced Changes in Serum Thyroid Hormones and Thyrotropin." *Metabolism* 27 (1978): 935–42.

Balsam, A. "The Influence of Fasting, Diabetes, and Several Pharmacological Agents on the Pathways of Thyroxine Metabolism in Rat Liver." *Journal of Clinical Investigation* 62 (1978): 415–24.

Banfalvi, Gaspar. *Heavy Metals, Trace Elements and Their Cellular Effects.* Boston, Mass.: Springer, 2011.

Basha, P. M., et al. "Fluoride Toxicity and Status of Serum Thyroid Hormones, Brain Histopathology, and Learning Memory in Rats: A Multigenerational Assessment." *Biological Trace Element Research* 144 (2011): 1083–94.

Beard, J. L., et al. "Impaired Thermoregulation and Thyroid Function in Iron-Deficiency Anemia." *American Journal of Clinical Nutrition* 52, no. 5 (1990): 813–19.

Becker, R. A., et al. "Free T4, Free T3 and Reverse T3 in Critically Ill, Thermally Injured Patients." *Journal of Trauma* 9 (1980).

Berson, S. A., and R. S. Yalow. "The Effect of Cortisone on the Iodine Accumulating Function of the Thyroid Gland in Euthyroid Subjects." *Journal of Clinical Endocrinology & Metabolism* 12 (1952): 407–22.

Bhatia, J., and F. Greer. "Use of Soy Protein-Based Formulas in Infant Feeding." *Pediatrics* 121 (2008): 148.

Biondi, B., and D. S. Cooper. "The Clinical Significance of Subclinical Thyroid Dysfunction." *Endocrine Reviews* 29 (2008): 76–131.

Boas, M., et al. "Environmental Chemicals and Thyroid Function." *European Journal of Endocrinology* 154 (2006): 599–611.

Bobek, S., et al. "Effect of Long-Term Fluoride Administration on Thyroid Hormones Level Blood in Rats." *Endocrinologia Experimentalis* 10 (1976): 289–95.

Bogoroch, R., and P. Timiras. "The Response of the Thyroid Gland of the Rat to Severe Stress." *Endocrinology* 49 (1951): 548–56.

Bondy, P. K., and M. A. Hagewood. "The Effect of Stress and Cortisone on Plasma Protein-Bound Iodine and Thyroxine Metabolism in Rats." *Proceedings of the Society for Experimental Biology and Medicine* 81, no. 1 (1952): 328–31.

Bosch, J., et al. "N-3 Fatty Acids and Cardiovascular Outcomes in Patients with Dysglycemia." *New England Journal of Medicine* 367 (2012): 1760–61.

Bouaziz, H., et al. "Effect of Fluoride Ingested by Lactating Mice on the Thyroid Function and Bone Maturation of Their Suckling Pups." *Fluoride* 2 (2004): 133–42.

Bozkurt, N., et al. "The Association between the Severity of Vitamin D Deficiency and Hashimoto's." *Endocrine Practice* 19 (2013): 479–84.

Brasky, T. M., et al. "Plasma Phospholipid Fatty Acids and Prostate Cancer Risk in the SELECT Trial." *Journal of the National Cancer Institute* 105 (2013): 1132–41.

Brown-Grant, K. "The Effect of Emotional and Physical Stress on Thyroid Activity in the Rabbit." *Journal of Physiology* 126 (1954): 29–40.

Brown-Grant, K. "The Influence of the Adrenal Cortex on Thyroid Activity in the Rabbit." *Journal of Physiology* 126 (1954): 41–51.

Brown-Grant, K., and G. Pethes. "The Response of the Thyroid Gland of the Guinea-Pig to Stress." *Journal of Physiology* 151 (1960): 40–50.

Brucker-Davis, F. "Effects of Environmental Synthetic Chemicals on Thyroid Function." *Thyroid* (1998): 827–56.

Burger, A., et al. "Reduced Active Thyroid Hormone Levels in Acute Illness." *Lancet* 1, no. 7961 (1976): 653–55.

Burgi, H., et al. "Changes of Circulating Thyroxine, Triiodothyronine and Reverse Triiodothyronine after Radiographic Contrast Agents." *Journal of Clinical Endocrinology & Metabolism* 43 (1976): 1203–10.

Burman, K. D., et al. "The Effect of T3 and Reverse T3 Administration on Muscle Protein Catabolism during Fasting as Measured by 3-methylhistidine Excretion." *Metabolism* 28 (1979): 805–13.

Burman, K. D., et al. "A Radioimmunoassay for 3,3',5'-L-Triiodothyronine (Reverse T3): Assessment of Thyroid Gland Content and Serum Measurements in Conditions of Normal and Altered Thyroidal Economy and Following Administration of Thyrotropin Releasing Hormone (TRH) and Thyrotropin (TSH)." *Journal of Clinical Endocrinology & Metabolism* 44 (1977): 660–72.

Burr, M. L., et al. "Lack of Benefit of Dietary Advice to Men with Angina: Results of a Controlled Trial." *European Journal of Clinical Nutrition* 57 (2003): 193–200.

Carter, J. N., et al. "Effect of Severe, Chronic Illness on Thyroid Function." *Lancet* 304 (1974): 971–74.

Cavalieri, R. R., and B. Rapoport. "Impaired Peripheral Conversion of Thyroxine to Triiodothyronine." *Annual Review of Medicine* 28 (1977): 57–65.

Chappell, L. T. "Applications of EDTA Chelation Therapy." *Alternative Medicine Review* 2 (1997): 426.

Chopra, I. J. "Assessment of Daily Production and Significance of Thyroidal Secretion of Reverse T3 in Man." *Journal of Clinical Investigation* 58 (1976): 32–40.

Chopra, I. J. "Misleadingly Low Free Thyroxine Index and Usefulness of Reverse Triiodothyronine Measurement in Nonthyroidal Illnesses." *Annals of Internal Medicine* 990 (1979): 905–12.

Chuong, C. M., et al. "What Is the 'True' Function of the Skin?" *Experimental Dermatology* 11 (2002): 159–87.

Cinemre, H., et al. "Hematologic Effects of Levothyroxine in Iron-Deficient Subclinical Hypothyroid Patients." *Journal of Clinical Endocrinology & Metabolism* 94 (2009): 151–56.

Cody, J. "Link between Fish Oil and Increased Risk of Colon Cancer in Mice." *MedicalNewsToday,* October 7, 2010. www.medicalnewstoday.com/releases/203683.php#post.

Collins, C. "Women with Type 1 Diabetes Receive No Heart Benefit from Omega-3." *MedicalNewsToday,* June 28, 2010. www.medicalnewstoday.com/releases/193107.php.

Contempre, B., et al. "Effects of Selenium Deficiency on Thyroid Necrosis, Fibrosis and Proliferation: A Possible Role in Myxoedematous Cretinism." *European Journal of Endocrinology* 133 (1995): 99–109.

Corvilain, B., et al. "Selenium and the Thyroid: How the Relationship Was Established." *American Journal of Clinical Nutrition* 57 (1993): 244S–48S.

D'Adamo, C. R. "Soy Foods and Supplementation: A Review of Commonly Perceived Health Benefits and Risks." *Alternative Therapies in Health Medicine* 20 (2014): 39–51.

D'Angelo, S. A. "Pituitary Regulation of Thyroid Gland Function" *Brookhaven Symposia in Biology* 7 (1955).

D'Aurizio, F., et al. "Is Vitamin D a Player or Not in the Pathophysiology of Autoimmune Thyroid Diseases?" *Autoimmunity Reviews* 14 (2015): 363–69.

Danforth, E., and A. G. Burger. "The Impact of Nutrition on Thyroid Hormone Physiology and Action." *Annual Review of Nutrition* 9 (1989): 201–27.

Danforth, E., et al. "Dietary-Induced Alterations in Thyroid Hormone Metabolism during Overnutrition." *Journal of Clinical Investigation* 64 (1979): 1336–47.

DeLemos, M. L. "Effects of Soy Phytoestrogens Genistein and Daidzein on Breast Cancer Growth." *Annals of Pharmacotherapeutics* 35 (2001): 1118–21.

DeLuca, H. F. "Vitamin D: The Vitamin and the Hormone." *Federation Proceedings* 33 (1974): 2211–19.

Demole, V. "Toxic Effects on the Thyroid." In *Fluorides and Human Health, Monograph Series* no. 59. Geneva: World Health Organization, 1970.

Dimich, A., et al. "Magnesium Transport in Patients with Thyroid Disease." *Journal of Clinical Endocrinology & Metabolism* 26 (1966): 1081–92.

Divia, R. L., et al. "Anti-thyroid Isoflavones from Soybean: Isolation, Characterization, and Mechanisms of Action." *Biochemical Pharmacology* 54 (1997): 1087–96.

Doerge, D., and D. Sheehan. "New Findings on the Soy/Thyroid Connection," *Thyroid-Info* 110, 3 (2002): 349–53.

Drutel, A., et al. "Selenium and the Thyroid Gland: More Good News For Clinicians." *Clinical Endocrinology* 78 (2013): 155–64.

Duntas, L. H., et al. "Incidence of Sideropenia and Effects of Iron Repletion Treatment in Women with Subclinical Hypothyroidism." *Experimental and Clinical Endocrinology & Diabetes* 107 (1999): 356–60.

Eales, J. G. "The Influence of Nutritional State on Thyroid Function in Various Vertebrates." *Integrative & Comparative Biology* 28 (1988): 351–62.

Ebling, F. John. *Hormonal Control of Mammalian Skin Glands.* Boston, Mass.: Springer, 1977.

Eftekhari, M. H., et al. "The Relationship Between Iron Status and Thyroid Hormone Concentration in Iron-Deficient Adolescent Iranian Girls." *Asia Pacific Journal of Clinical Nutrition* 15 (2006): 50–55.

Engstrom, W. W., and B. Markardt. "The Effects of Serious Illness and Surgical Stress on the Circulating Thyroid Hormone." *Journal of Clinical Endocrinology & Metabolism* 15 (1955): 953–63.

Ericsson, U. B., et al. "Effects of Cigarette Smoking on Thyroid Function and the Prevalence of Goitre, Thyrotoxicosis and Autoimmune Thyroiditis." *Journal of Internal Medicine* 229 (1991): 67–71.

Faccini, J. M., et al. "Effect of Sodium Fluoride on the Ultrastructure of the Parathyroid Gland of Sheep." *Nature* 207 (1965): 1399–401.

Farbridge, K. J., et al. "Temporal Effects of Restricted Diet and Compensatory Increased Dietary Intake on Thyroid Function, Plasma Growth Hormone Levels and Tissue Lipid Reserves of Rainbow Trout." *Aquaculture* 104 (1992): 157–74.

Farquharson, A. L., et al. "Effect of Dietary Fish Oil on Atrial Fibrillation after Cardiac Surgery." *American Journal of Cardiology* (2011): 851–56.

Fein, H. G., et al. "Anemia in Thyroid Diseases." *Medical Clinics of North America* 59 (1975): 1133–45.

Fitzpatrick, M. "Soy Formulas and the Effects of Isoflavones on the Thyroid." *New Zealand Medical Journal* 113 (2000): 24–26.

Fontana, L., et al. "Effect of Long-Term Calorie Restriction with Adequate Protein and Micronutrients on Thyroid Hormones." *Journal of Clinical Endocrinology & Metabolism* 91 (2006): 3232–35.

Furr, M. O., et al. "The Effects of Stress on Gastric Ulceration, T3, T4, Reverse T3 and Cortisol in Neonatal Foals." *Equine Veterinary Journal* 24 (1992): 37–40.

Galan, P., et al. "Effects of B Vitamins and Omega 3 Fatty Acids on Cardiovascular Diseases." *British Medical Journal* 341 (2010): 6273.

Galetti, P. M., and G. Joyet. "Effect of Fluorine on Thyroidal Iodine Metabolism in Hyperthyroidism." *Journal of Clinical Endocrinology & Metabolism* 18, no. 10 (1958): 1102–10.

Gavin, L., et al. "Extrathyroidal Conversion of Thyroxine to 3,3',5'-Triiodothyronine (Reverse T3) and to 3,5,3'- Triiodothyronine." *Journal of Clinical Endocrinology & Metabolism* 44 (1977): 733–42.

Gedalia, I., et al. "The Effects of Water Fluorination on Thyroid Function, Bones and Teeth of Rats on a Low Iodine Diet." *Archives of Internal Pharmacodynamics & Therapeutics* 129 (1960): 312–15.

Georgiou, G. J. "The Discovery of A Unique Natural Heavy Metal Chelator." *Explore!* 14 (2005): 1–8.

Gerwing, J., et al. "The Influence of Bacterial Exotoxins on the Activity of the Thyroid Gland in Different Species." *Journal of Physiology* 144 (1958): 229–42.

Ginsberg, J., et al. "Cord Blood Reverse T3 in Normal, Premature, Euthyroid Low T4 and Hypothyroid Newborns." *Journal of Endocrinological Investigation* 1 (1978): 73–77.

Goswami, R., et al. "Prevalence of Vitamin D Deficiency and Its Relationship with Thyroid Autoimmunity in Asian Indians: A Community Based Survey." *British Journal of Nutrition* 102 (2009): 382–86.

Greenberg, N., and J. C. Wingfield. "Stress and Reproduction: Reciprocal Relationships." In *Hormones and Reproduction in Fishes, Amphibians, and Reptiles,* 461–503. Boston, Mass.: Springer, 1987.

Griffiths, R. S., et al. "Measurement of Serum 3,3'5'- (Reverse) T3, with Comments on Its Derivation." *Clinical Endocrinology* 5 (1976): 679–85.

Hall, R., et al. "The Thyrotropin-Releasing Hormone Test in Diseases of the Pituitary and Hypothalamus." *Lancet* 299 (1972): 759–63.

Harris, A. R. C. "Effect of Starvation, Nutriment Replacement, and Hypothyroidism on In Vitro Hepatic T4 to T3 Conversion in the Rat." *Metabolism* 27 (1978): 1680–90.

Harwood, J. "The Adipocyte as an Endocrine Organ in the Regulation of Metabolic Homeostasis." *Neuropharmacology* 63 (2012): 57–75.

Heimreich, D. L., et al. "Relationship between the Hypothalamic-Pituitary-Thyroid (HPT) Axis and the Hypothalamic-Pituitary-Adrenal (HPA) Axis during Repeated Stress." *Neuroendocrinology* 81 (2005): 183–92.

Herlihy, J. T., et al. "Long Term Food Restriction Depresses Serum Thyroid Hormone Concentrations in the Rat." *Mechanisms of Ageing and Development* 53 (1990): 9–16.

Hesch, R. D., et al. "Conversion of Thyroxine (T4) and Triiodothyronine (T3) and the Subcellular Localisation of the Converting Enzyme." *Clinical Chimica Acta* 59 (1975): 209–13.

Hill, J. O., et al. "Environmental Contributions to the Obesity Epidemic." *Science* 280 (1998): 1371–74.

Hy, R. A., et al. "The Therapeutic Effect of Combined Aqueous Extract of Coriander Sativum L. and Allium Sativum L. on the Mercuric Chloride Induced Reproductive Toxicity in Adult Male Rats." *Basrah Journal of Veterinary Research* 12 (2013): 185–202.

Ingbar, S. H., and L. E. Braverman. "Active Form of the Thyroid Hormone." *Annual Review of Medicine* 26 (1975): 1–601.

Jabbar, A., et al. "Vitamin B₁₂ Deficiency Common in Primary Hypothyroidism." *Journal of the Pakistan Medical Association* 58 (2008): 258–61.

Jabbar, M. A., et al. "Abnormal Thyroid Function Tests in Infants with Congenital Hypothyroidism: The Influence of Soy-Based Formula." *Journal of the American College of Nutrition* 16 (1997): 280–82.

James, P. T., et al. "The Worldwide Obesity Epidemic." *Obesity* 9 (2001): 2285–335.

Jennings, A. S., et al. "Regulation of the Conversion of Thyroxine to Triiodothyronine in the Perfused Rat Liver." *Journal of Clinical Investigation* 64 (1979): 1614–23.

Jones, J. E., et al. "Magnesium Metabolism in Hyperthyroidism and Hypothyroidism." *Journal of Clinical Investigation* 45 (1966): 891–900.

Kahn, Mara. *Vegan Betrayal.* Boulder, Colo.: Little Boat Press, 2016.

Kansal, L., et al. "Protective Role of Coriandrum sativum (Coriander) Extracts against Lead Nitrate Induced Oxidative Stress and Tissue Damage in the Liver and Kidney in Male Mice." *International Journal of Applied Biology and Pharmaceutical Technology* 2, no. 3 (2011).

Kaplan, M. M., et al. "Changes in Serum Reverse T3 Concentrations with Altered Thyroid Hormone Secretion and Metabolism." *Journal of Clinical Endocrinology & Metabolism* 45 (2016): 447–56.

Kaplan, M. M., et al. "Changes in Serum 3,3',5'-Triiodothyronine (Reverse T3) Concentrations with Altered Thyroid Hormone Secretion and Metabolism." *Journal of Clinical Endocrinology & Metabolism* 45 (1977): 447–56.

Kaplan, M. M., et al. "Prevalence of Abnormal Thyroid Function Test Results in Patients with Acute Medical Illnesses." *American Journal of Medicine* 72 (1982): 9–16.

Kioukia-Fougia, N., et al. "The Effects of Stress Exposure on the Hypothalamic-Pituitary-Adrenal Axis, Thymus, Thyroid Hormones and Glucose Levels." *Progress in Neuro-Psychopharmacology and Biological Psychiatry* 26 (2002): 823–30.

Kivity, S., et al. "Vitamin D and Autoimmune Thyroid Diseases." *Cellular & Molecular Immunology* 8 (2011): 243–48.

Klein, A. H., et al. "Cord Blood Reverse T3 in Congenital Hypothyroidism." *Journal of Clinical Endocrinology & Metabolism* 46 (1978): 336–38.

Knobeloch, L., et al. "Methylmercury Exposure in Wisconsin: A Case Study Series." *Environmental Research* 101 (2006): 113–22.

Kowey, P. R., et al. "Efficacy and Safety of Prescription Omega-3 Fatty Acids for the Prevention of Recurrent Symptomatic Atrial Fibrillation." *Journal of the American Medical Association* 304 (2010): 2363–72.

Kromhout, D., et al. "N-3 Fatty Acids and Cardiovascular Events after Myocardial Infarction." *New England Journal of Medicine* 363 (2010): 2015–26.

Kvetny, J., et al. "Subclinical Hypothyroidism Is Associated with a Low-Grade Inflammation, Increased Triglyceride Levels and Predicts Cardiovascular Disease in Males below 50 Years." *Clinical Endocrinology* 61 (2004): 232–38.

Labib, M., et al. "Dietary Maladvice as a Cause of Hypothyroidism and Short Stature." *British Medical Journal* 298 (1989): 232–33.

Lands, W. E. M., et al. "Quantitative Effects of Dietary Polyunsaturated Fats on the Composition of Fatty Acids in Rat Tissue." *Lipids* (1990): 505–51.

Laurberg, P., et al. "Environmental Iodine Intake Affects the Type of Nonmalignant Thyroid Disease." *Thyroid* 11 (2001): 457–69.

Laurberg, P., et al. "High Incidence of Multinodular Toxic Goitre in the Elderly Population in a Low Iodine Intake Area vs. High Incidence of Graves' Disease in the Young in a High Iodine Intake Area: Comparative Surveys of Thyrotoxicosis Epidemiology in East-Jutland Denmark and Iceland." *Journal of Internal Medicine* 229 (1991): 415–20.

Leung, A. M., et al. "Iodine Status and Thyroid Function of Boston-Area Vegetarians and Vegans." *Journal of Clinical Endocrinology & Metabolism* 96 (2011): E1303–7.

Lightner, E. S., et al. "Intra-amniotic Injection of Thyroxine (T4) to a Human Fetus: Evidence for Conversion of T4 to Reverse T3." *American Journal of Obstetrics and Gynecology* 127 (1977): 487–90.

Mackawy, A. M. H., et al. "Vitamin D Deficiency and Its Association with Thyroid Disease." *International Journal of Health Sciences* 7 (2013): 267–75.

Makrides, M., et al. "Effect of DHA Supplementation during Pregnancy on Maternal Depression and Neurodevelopment of Young Children." *Journal of the American Medical Association* 304 (2010): 1675–83.

Malyszko, J., et al. "Thyroid Function, Endothelium, and Inflammation in Hemodialyzed Patients: Possible Relations?" *Journal of Renal Nutrition* 17 (2007): 30–37.

Mason, R. P., et al. "Omega-3 Fatty Acid Fish Oil Dietary Supplements Contain Saturated Fats and Oxidized Lipids That May Interfere with Their Intended Biological Benefits." *Biochemical and Biophysical Research Communications* 483 (2017): 425–29.

Mastorakos, G., and M. Paviatou. "Exercise as a Stress Model and the Interplay between the Hypothalamus-Pituitary-Adrenal and the Hypothalamus-Pituitary-Thyroid Axes." *Hormone and Metabolic Research* 37 (2005): 577–84.

McGown, C., et al. "Adipose Tissue as an Endocrine Organ." *Clinics in Liver Disease* 18 (2014): 41–58.

Mehmet, E., et al. "Characteristics of Anemia in Subclinical and Overt Hypothyroid Patients." *Endocrine Journal* 59 (2012): 213–20.

Messina, M. "Effects of Soy Protein and Soybean Isoflavones on Thyroid Function in Healthy Adults and Hypothyroid Patients." *Thyroid* 16 (2006): 249–58.

Michalaki, M. A., et al. "Thyroid Function in Humans with Morbid Obesity." *Thyroid* 16 (2006): 73–78.

Mizokami, T., et al. "Stress and Thyroid Autoimmunity." *Thyroid* 14 (2004): 1047–55.

Mokdad, A. H., et al. "The Spread of the Obesity Epidemic in the United States, 1991–1998." *Journal of the American Medical Association* 2892 (1999): 1519–22.

Morley, J. E., et al. "Zinc Deficiency, Chronic Starvation and Hypothalamic-Pituitary-Thyroid Function." *American Journal of Clinical Nutrition* 33 (1980): 1767–70.

Mozaffarian, D., et al. "Fish Oil and Postoperative Atrial Fibrillation: The Omega-3 Fatty Acids for Prevention of Post-Operative Atrial Fibrillation (OPERA) Randomized Trial." *Journal of the American Medical Association* 308 (2012): 2001–11.

Neustaedter, R. "Soy Unsafe for Children." In *Child Health Guide: Pediatrics for Parents,* 51–53. Berkeley, Calif.: North Atlantic Books, 2005.

Ober, Clinton, Stephen T. Sinatra, and Martin Zucker. *Earthing.* Columbus, Ohio: Basic Health Publications, 2014.

Olney, R. S., et al. "Prevalence of Congenital Hypothyroidism—Current Trends and Future Directions." Workshop Summary. *Pediatrics* 125 (2010).

Pandey, S. "Chelation Therapy and Chelating Agents of Ayurveda." International *Journal of Green Pharmacy* 10, no. 3 (2016): 143–50.

Passos, M. C. F., et al. "Long-Term Effects of Malnutrition during Lactation on the Thyroid Function of Offspring." *Hormone and Metabolic Research* 34 (2002): 40–43.

Pearce, E. N., et al. "Environmental Pollutants and the Thyroid." *Best Practice & Research: Clinical Endocrinology & Metabolism* 23 (2009): 801–13.

Pinchera, A., et al. "Thyroid Refractoriness in an Athyreotic Cretin Fed Soybean Formula." *New England Journal of Medicine* 273 (1965): 83–87.

Poncin, S., et al. "Oxidative Stress in the Thyroid Gland: From Harmlessness to Hazard Depending on the Iodine Content." *Endocrinology* 149 (2008): 424–33.

Pot, G. K. "No Effects of Fish Oil Supplementation on Serum Inflammatory Markers and Their Interrelationships." *European Journal of Clinical Nutrition* 62 (2009): 1353–50.

Potter, S. "Soy Protein and Cardiovascular Disease: The Impact of Bioactive Components in Soy." *Nutrition Reviews* 56 (2014): 231–35.

Redding, J. M., et al. "Cortisol and Its Effects on Plasma Thyroid Hormone and Electrolyte Concentrations in Fresh Water and During Seawater Acclimation in Yearling Coho Salmon." *General and Comparative Endocrinology* 56 (1984): 146–55.

Rizos, E. C., et al. "Association between Omega-3 Fatty Acid Supplementation and Risk of Major Cardiovascular Disease Events." *Journal of the American Medical Association* 308 (2012): 1024–33.

Robbins, J. "Factors Altering Thyroid Hormone Metabolism." *Environmental Health Perspectives* 38 (1981): 65–70.

Rolland, R. M. "A Review of Chemically-Induced Alterations in Thyroid and Vitamin A Status from Field Studies of Wildlife and Fish." *Journal of Wildlife Diseases* 36 (2000): 615–35.

Roosterman, D., et al. "Neuronal Control of Skin Function: The Skin as a Neuroimmunoendocrine Organ." *Physiological Reviews* 86 (2006): 1309–79.

Sacks, F., et al. "Controlled Trial of Fish Oil for Regression of Coronary Atherosclerosis." *Journal of the American College of Cardiology* 25 (1995): 1492–98.

Sathyapalan, T., et al. "The Effect of Soy Phytoestrogen Supplementation on Thyroid Status and Cardiovascular Risk Markers in Patients with Subclinical Hypothyroidism." *Journal of Clinical Endocrinology & Metabolism* 96 (2011): 1442–49.

Sears, M. E. "Chelation: Harnessing and Enhancing Heavy Metal Detoxification." *Scientific World Journal* 2013 (2013).

Shin, D. Y., et al. "Low Serum Vitamin D Is Associated with Anti-thyroid Peroxidase Antibody in Autoimmune Thyroiditis." *Yonsei Medical Journal* 55 (2014): 476–81.

Simao, A. N., et al. "[Effect of n-3 Fatty Acids in Glycemic and Lipid Profiles, Oxidative Stress and Total Antioxidant Capacity in Patients with the Metabolic Syndrome]" (article in Portuguese). *Arquivos Brasileiros de Endocrinologia & Metabologia* 54, no. 5(2010): 463–69.

Simao, A. N., et al. "Effect of Soy Product Kinako and Fish Oil on Serum Lipids and Glucose Metabolism in Women with Metabolic Syndrome." *Nutrition* 30 (2014): 112–15.

Singh, A., et al. "Reduction of Heavy Metal Load in Food Chain: Technology Assessment." *Reviews in Environmental Science and Bio/Technology* 10 (2011): 199.

Slominski, A., et al. "Skin as an Endocrine Organ: Implications for Its Function." *Drug Discovery Today: Disease Mechanisms* 5 (2008): 137–44.

Soslc-Jurjevic, B., et al. "Soy Isoflavones Interfere with Thyroid Hormone Homeostasis." *Toxicology and Applied Pharmacology* 278 (2014): 124–34.

Spaulding, S. W., et al. "Effect of Caloric Restriction and Dietary Composition on Serum T3 and Reverse T3 in Man." *Journal of Clinical Endocrinology & Metabolism* 42 (2016): 197–200.

Stacpoole, P., et al. "Effects of Dietary Marine Oil on Carbohydrate and Lipid Metabolism in Normal Subjects and Patients with Hypertriglyceridemia." *Metabolism* 38 (1989): 946–56.

Surks, M. I., et al. "Subclinical Thyroid Disease: Scientific Review and Guidelines for Diagnosis and Management." *Journal of the American Medical Association* 291 (2004): 228–38.

Susheela, A. K., et al. "Excess Fluoride Ingestion and Thyroid Hormone Derangements in Children Living in Delhi, India." *Fluoride* 38 (2005): 98–108.

Szkudelska, K., et al. "Genistein—A Dietary Compound Inducing Hormonal and Metabolic Changes." *Journal of Steroid Biochemistry and Molecular Biology* 105 (2007): 37–45.

Tamer, G., et al. "Relative Vitamin D Insufficiency in Hashimoto's Thyroiditis." *Thyroid* 21 (2011): 891–96.

Teng, W., et al. "Effect of Iodine Intake on Thyroid Diseases in China." *New England Journal of Medicine* 354 (2006): 2783–93.

Thiboutot, D., et al. "Human Skin Is a Steroidogenic Tissue: Steroidogenic Enzymes and Cofactors Are Expressed in Epidermis, Normal Sebocytes, and an Immortalized Sebocyte Cell Line." *Journal of Investigative Dermatology* 120 (2003): 905–14.

Thuppil, V., et al. "Treating Lead Toxicity: Possibilities beyond Synthetic Chelation." *Journal of Krishna Institute of Medical Sciences University* 2 (2013): 4–31.

Tilg, H., et al. "Evolution of Inflammation in Nonalcoholic Fatty Liver Disease: The Multiple Parallel Hits Hypothesis." *Hepatology* 52 (2010): 1836–46.

Tilg, H., et al. "Insulin Resistance, Inflammation and Non-alcoholic Fatty Liver Disease." *Trends in Endocrinology & Metabolism* 19 (2008): 371–79.

Tomimori, E., et al. "Prevalence of Incidental Thyroid Disease in a Relatively Low Iodine Intake Area." *Thyroid* 5 (1995): 273–76.

Trabelsi, M., et al. "Effect of Fluoride on Thyroid Function and Cerebellar Development in Mice." *Fluoride* 34 (2001): 165–73.

Trenev, N. *Probiotics: Nature's Internal Healers.* New York: Avery, 1998.

Tsatsoulis, A. "The Role of Stress in the Clinical Expression of Thyroid Autoimmunity." *Neuroendocrine and Immune Crosstalk* 1088 (2006): 382–95.

Tudhope, G. R., et al. "Deficiency of Vitamin B12 in Hypothyroidism." *Lancet* 7 (1962): 703–6.

Turker, O., et al. "Selenium Treatment in Autoimmune Thyroiditis: 9-Month Follow-up with Variable Doses." *Journal of Endocrinology* 190 (2006): 151–56.

Vazquez-Vela, Maria Eugenia Frigolet, et al. "White Adipose Tissue as Endocrine Organ and Its Role in Obesity." *Archives of Medical Research* 39 (2008): 715–28.

Veirord, M. B., et al. "Diet and Risk of Cutaneous Malignant Melanoma: A Prospective Study of 50,757 Norwegian Men and Women." *International Journal of Cancer* 71 (1997): 600–604.

Von Schacky, C., et al. "The Effect of Dietary-3 Fatty Acids on Coronary Atherosclerosis." *Annals of Internal Medicine* 130 (1999): 554–62.

Wainwright, P. E., et al. "The Effects of Dietary n-3/n-6 Ratio on Brain Development in the Mouse: A Dose Response Study with Long Chain n-3 Fatty Acids." *Lipids* 27 (1992): 98–103.

Walz, C. P., et al. "Omega-3 polyunsaturated Fatty Acid Supplementation in the Prevention of Cardiovascular Disease." *Canadian Pharmaceutical Journal* 149 (2016): 166–73.

Wang, H., et al. "Fluoride-Induced Thyroid Dysfunction in Rats: Roles of Dietary Protein and Calcium Level." *Toxicology and Industrial Health* 9 (2009): 105–16.

Wang, Y., and M. A. Beydoun. "The Obesity Epidemic in the United States— Gender, Age, Socioeconomic, Racial/Ethnic, and Geographic Characteristics." *Epidemiologic Reviews* 29 (2007): 6–28.

Williams, R. H., et al. "Effect of Severe Stress upon Thyroid Function." *American Journal of Physiology* 159 (1949): 291–97.

Woodworth, H. L., et al. "Dietary Fish Oil Alters T-lymphocyte Cell Populations and Exacerbates Disease in a Mouse Model of Inflammatory Colitis." *Cancer Research* 70 (2010): 7960–69.

Wozniak, S. E., et al. "Adipose Tissue: The New Endocrine Organ?" *Digestive Diseases and Sciences* 54 (2009): 1847–56.

Yasuda, T., et al. "Serum Vitamin D Levels Are Decreased and Associated with Thyroid Volume in Female Patients with Newly Onset Graves' Disease." *Endocrine* 42 (2012): 739–41.

Zhan, X., et al. "Effects of Fluoride on Growth and Thyroid Function in Young Pigs." *Fluoride* 39 (2006): 95–100.

Zimmermann, M. B., et al. "Iron Deficiency Predicts Poor Maternal Thyroid Status during Pregnancy." *Journal of Clinical Endocrinology & Metabolism* 92 (2007): 3436–40.

Zimmermann, M. B., and J. Kohrle. "The Impact of Iron and Selenium Deficiencies on Iodine and Thyroid Metabolism: Biochemistry and Relevance to Public Health." *Thyroid* 12 (2002): 867–78.

Zouboulis, C. C. "The Human Skin as a Hormone Target and an Endocrine Gland." *Hormones* 3 (2004): 9–26.

Zouboulis, C. C. "The Skin as an Endocrine Organ." *Journal of Dermato-Endocrinology* 1 (2009): 250–52.

Zouboulis, C. C., et al. "Human Skin: An Independent Peripheral Endocrine Organ." *Hormone Research in Paediatrics* 54 (2000): 230–42.

Zouboulis, C. C., et al. "Sexual Hormones in Human Skin." *Hormone and Metabolic Research* 39 (2007): 85–95.

4. THYROID AND ADRENAL INTERACTIONS

Abalovich, M., et al. "Overt and Subclinical Hypothyroidism Complicating Pregnancy." *Thyroid* 12 (2002): 63–68.

Abrams, J. J., and S. M. Grundy. "Cholesterol Metabolism in Hypothyroidism and Hyperthyroidism in Man." *Journal of Lipid Research* 22 (1981): 323–38.

Abramson, J., "Thyroid Antibodies and Fetal Loss: An Evolving Story." *Thyroid* 11 (2001): 57–63.

Agarwal, R., et al. "Studies on Immunomodulatory Activity of Withania somnifera (Ashwagandha) Extracts in Experimental Immune Inflammation." *Journal of Ethnopharmacology* 67 (1999): 27–35.

Agdeppa, D., et al. "Plasma High Density Lipoprotein Cholesterol in Thyroid Disease." *Journal of Clinical Endocrinology & Metabolism* 49 (1979): 726–29.

Akpinar, S. "Restless Legs Syndrome Treatment with Dopaminergic Drugs." *Clinical Neuropharmacology* 10 (1987): 69–79.

Albright, F., et al. "Postmenopausal Osteoporosis: Its Clinical Features." *Journal of the American Medical Association* 116 (1941): 2465–74.

Allen, R. "Dopamine and Iron in the Pathophysiology of Restless Legs Syndrome." *Sleep Medicine* 4 (2004): 385–91.

Alnouti, Y. "Bile Acid Sulfation: A Pathway of Bile Acid Elimination and Detoxification." *Toxicology Science* 108 (2009): 225–46.

Althaus, B. U., et al. "LDL/HDL Changes in Subclinical Hypothyroidism: Possible Risk Factors for Coronary Heart Disease." *Clinical Endocrinology* 28 (1988): 157–63.

Baliram, R., et al. "Hyperthyroid-Associated Osteoporosis Is Exacerbated by the Loss of TSH Signaling." *Journal of Clinical Investigation* 10, no. 22 (2012): 3737–41.

Bartalena, L., et al. "Relationship of the Increased Serum Interleukin-6 Concentration to Changes of Thyroid Function in Nonthyroidal Illness." *Journal of Endocrinological Investigation* 17 (1994): 269–74.

Bartalena, L., et al. "Role of Cytokines in the Pathogenesis of the Euthyroid Sick Syndrome." *European Journal of Endocrinology* 138 (1998): 603-614.

Benhadi, N., et al. "Higher Maternal TSH Levels in Pregnancy Are Associated with Increased Risk for Miscarriage, Fetal or Neonatal Death." *European Journal of Endocrinology* 160 (2009): 985–91.

Bharucha, A. E., et al. "Slow Transit Constipation." *Gastroenterology Clinics of North America* 30 (2001): 77–96.

Bindels, A. J. G. H., et al. "The Prevalence of Subclinical Hypothyroidism at Different Total Plasma Levels in Middle Aged Men and Women: A Need for Case-Finding?" *Clinical Endocrinology* 50 (1999): 217–20.

Biondi, B., et al. "Hypothyroidism as a Risk Factor for Cardiovascular Disease." *Endocrine* 24 (2004): 1–13.

Birch, M. P., et al. "Female Pattern Hair Loss." *Clinical and Experimental Dermatology* 27 (2002): 383–88.

Boelen, A., et al. "Association between Serum Interleukin-6 and Serum 3,5,3'-Triiodothyronine in Nonthyroidal Illness." *Journal of Clinical & Endocrinological Metabolism* 77 (1993): 1695–99.

Boonstra, R. "Reality as the Leading Cause of Stress: Rethinking the Impact of Chronic Stress in Nature." *Functional Ecology* 27 (2013): 11–23.

Bopana, N., and S. Saxena. "In Vitro Propagation of High Value Medicinal Plant: Asparagus racemosus Willd." *Plant* 44 (2008): 525–32.

Brabant, G., et al. "Physiological Regulation of Circadian and Pulsatile Thyrotropin Secretion in Normal Man and Woman." *Journal of Clinical Endocrinology & Metabolism* 70 (1990): 403–9.

Braverman, L. E. "Iodine and the Thyroid: 33 Years of Study." *Thyroid* 4 (1994): 351–56.

Buysse, D. J. "Chronic Insomnia." *American Journal of Psychiatry* 165 (2008): 678–86.

Cann, S. A., et al. "Hypothesis: Iodine, Selenium and the Development of Breast Cancer." *Cancer Causes & Control* 11 (2000): 121–27.

Cappola, A. R., et al. "Hypothyroidism and Atherosclerosis." *Journal of Clinical Endocrinology & Metabolism* 88 (2003): 2438–44.

Casey, B. M., et al. "Subclinical Hypothyroidism and Pregnancy Outcomes." *Obstetrics & Gynecology* 105 (2005): 239–45.

Chahal, H. S., and W. M. Drake. "The Endocrine System and Ageing." *Journal of Pathology* 211 (2007): 173–80.

Chen, C. H., et al. "Congenital Hypothyroidism with Multiple Ovarian Cysts." *European Journal of Pediatrics* 158 (1999): 851–52.

Choksi, N. Y., et al. "Role of Thyroid Hormones in Human and Laboratory Animal Reproductive Health." *Developmental and Reproductive Toxicology* 68 (2003): 479–91.

Ciocon, J. O., et al. "Leg Edema: Clinical Clues to the Differential Diagnosis." *Geriatrics* 48 (1993): 34–45.

Cowan, L. D., et al. "Breast Cancer Incidence in Women with a History of Progesterone Deficiency." *American Journal of Epidemiology* 114 (1981): 209–17.

Das, S. K. "Tulsi: The Indian Holy Power Plant." *Indian Journal of Natural Products and Resources* 5 (2006): 279–83.

Davis, S. R., et al. "Endocrine Aspects of Female Sexual Dysfunction." *Journal of Sexual Medicine* 1 (2004): 82–86.

Dayan, C., et al. "Interpretation of Thyroid Function Tests." *Lancet* 357 (2001): 619–24.

Delitala, G. "Dopamine and TSH Secretion in Man." *Lancet* 310 (1977): 760–61.

Dendrinos, S., et al. "Thyroid Autoimmunity in Patients with Recurrent Spontaneous Miscarriages." *Gynecological Endocrinology* 14 (2000): 270–74.

Devasagayam, T. P. A., and K. B. Sainis. "Immune System and Antioxidants, Especially Those Derived from Indian Medicinal Plants." *Indian Journal of Experimental Biology* 40 (2002): 639–55.

Diekman, T., et al. "Prevalence and Correction of Hypothyroidism in a Large Cohort of Patients Referred for Dyslipidemia." *Archives of Internal Medicine* 155 (1995): 1490–95.

Dimich, A., et al. "Magnesium Transport in Patients with Thyroid Disease." *Journal of Clinical Endocrinology & Metabolism* 26 (2016): 1081–92.

Dittrich, Ralf, et al. "Thyroid Hormone Receptors and Reproduction." *Journal of Reproductive Immunology* 90 (2011): 58–66.

Douillard, J. "Shilajit." John Douillard's LifeSpa, http://lifespa.com/ayurvedic -supplement-facts/shilajit. Accessed September 2018.

Eastwood, G. L., et al. "Reversal of Lower Esophageal Sphincter Hypotension and Esophageal Aperistalsis after Treatment for Hypothyroidism." *Journal of Clinical Gastroenterology* 4, no. 4 (1982): 307–10.

Ebert, E. C. "The Thyroid and the Gut." *Journal of Clinical Gastroenterology* 44 (2010): 402–6.

Einarsson, K., et al. "Influence of Age on Secretion of Cholesterol and Synthesis of Bile Acids by the Liver." *New England Journal of Medicine* 313 (1985): 277–82.

Elder, J., et al. "The Relationship between Serum Cholesterol and Serum Thyrotropin, Thyroxine and Triiodothyronine Concentrations in Suspected Hypothyroidism." *Annals of Clinical Biochemistry: International Journal of Laboratory Medicine* 27 (1990): 110–13.

Ely, J. W., et al. "Approach to Leg Edema of Unclear Etiology." *Journal of the American Board of Family Medicine* 19 (2006): 148–60.

Fajer, A. B., et al. "The Contribution of the Adrenal Gland to the Total Amount of Progesterone Produced in the Female Rate." *Journal of Physiology* 214 (1971): 115–26.

Feek, C. M., et al. "Influence of Thyroid Status on Dopaminergic Inhibition of Thyrotropin and Prolactin Secretion: Evidence for an Additional Feedback Mechanism in the Control of Thyroid Hormone Secretion." *Journal of Clinical Endocrinology & Metabolism* 51 (1980): 585–89.

Field, T., and M. Diego. "Cortisol: The Culprit Prenatal Stress Variable." *International Journal of Neuroscience* 118 (2008): 1181–205.

Ford, H. B., and D. J. Schust. "Recurrent Pregnancy Loss: Etiology, Diagnosis and Therapy." *Review of Obstetrics and Gynecology* 2 (2009): 76–83.

Fredlund, B., and S. B. Olsson. "Long QT Interval and Ventricular Tachycardia of 'Torsade de Pointe' Type in Hypothyroidism." *Journal of Internal Medicine* 213 (1983): 231–35.

Freedberg, A. S., et al. "The Effect of Altered Thyroid State on Atrial Intracellular Potentials." *Journal of Physiology* 207 (1970): 357–69.

Freinkel, R. K., and N. Freinkel. "Hair Growth and Alopecia in Hypothyroidism." *Archives of Dermatology* 106 (1972): 349–52.

Frizel, D., et al. "Plasma Levels of Ionised Calcium and Magnesium in Thyroid Disease." *Lancet* 1, no. 7504 (1967): 1360–61.

Fudge, J. R., et al. "Medical Evaluation for Exposure Extremes: Cold." *Clinical Journal of Sport Medicine* 26 (2015): 63–68.

Fukuda, K., et al. "The Chronic Fatigue Syndrome: A Comprehensive Approach to Its Definition and Study." *Annals of Internal Medicine* 121 (1994): 953–59.

Ghaemi, N., et al. "Delayed Diagnosis of Hypothyroidism in Children." *Iranian Red Crescent Medical Journal* 17 (2015): e20306.

Gidley-Baird, A., et al. "Failure of Implantation in Human In Vitro Fertilization and Embryo Transfer Patients: The Effects of Altered Progesterone/Estrogen Ratios in Humans and Mice." *Fertility and Sterility* 45 (1986): 69–74.

Glinoer, D., et al. "Risk of Subclinical Hypothyroidism in Pregnant Women with Asymptomatic Autoimmune Thyroid Disorders." *Journal of Clinical Endocrinology & Metabolism* 79 (1994): 197–204.

Gold, M. S., et al. "Hypothyroidism and Depression: Evidence from Complete Thyroid Function Evaluation." *Journal of the American Medical Association* 245 (1981): 1919–22.

Goyal, R. K., et al. "Asparagus racemosus—An Update." *Indian Journal of Medical Sciences* 57, no. 9 (2003): 408–13.

Grandhi, A., et al. "A Comparative Pharmacological Investigation of Ashwagandha and Ginseng." *Journal of Ethnopharmacology* 44 (1994): 131–35.

Gurkan, S., et al. "A Case of Autoimmune Thyroiditis and Mebranoproliferative Glomerulonephritis." *Pediatric Nephrology* 24 (2009): 193–97.

Gussekloo, J., et al. "Thyroid Status, Disability and Cognitive Function and Survival in Old Age." *Journal of the American Medical Association* 292 (2004): 2591–99.

Hage, M., et al. "Thyroid Disorders and Diabetes Mellitus." *Journal of Thyroid Research* 2011 (2011). doi:10.4061/2011/439463.

Hakkim, F. L., et al. "Chemical Composition and Antioxidant Property of Holy Basil (Ocimum sanctum L.) Leaves, Stems and Inflorescence and Their In Vitro Callus Cultures." *Journal of Agricultural and Food Chemistry* 55 (2007): 9109–17.

Hall, D. C. "Nutritional Influences on Estrogen Metabolism." *Applied Nutritional Science Reports* 1 (2001).

Harbison, J. "Sleep Disorders in Older People." *Age and Ageing* 31, suppl. 2 (2002): 6–9.

Hecht, A., et al. "Diabetes Mellitus and Primary Hypothyroidism." *Metabolism* 17 (1968): 108–13.

Heeringa, J., et al. "High-Normal Thyroid Function and Risk of Atrial Fibrillation." *Archives of Internal Medicine* 168 (2008): 2219–24.

Hein, M. D., et al. "Thyroid Function in Psychiatric Illness." *General Hospital Psychiatry* 12 (1990): 232–44.

Hermann, P. T., et al. "Forskolin: From an Ayurvedic Remedy to a Modern Agent." *Planta Medica* 51 (1989): 473–77.

Hodgson, H., and R. Malik. "The Relationship between the Thyroid Gland and the Liver." *Quarterly Journal of Medicine* 95 (2002): 559–69.

Idzikowski, C., and C. M. Shapiro. "ABC of Sleep Disorders. Non-Psychotropic Drugs and Sleep." *British Medical Journal* 306 (1993): 1118–21.

Iglesias, P., and J. J. Diez. "Thyroid Dysfunction and Kidney Disease." *Endocrinology* 160 (2009): 503–15.

Jackson, M. D. "The Thyroid Axis and Depression." Thyroid 8 (1998): 951–56.

Jain, S., and G. S. Jogad. "Role of Ayurvedic Management in Post Natal Hypothyroidism." *Journal of Indian System of Medicine* 3, no. 4 (2015): 209–13.

Joffe, B. I., and L. A. Distiller. "Diabetes Mellitus and Hypothyroidism: Strange Bedfellows or Mutual Companions?" *World Journal of Diabetes* 5 (2014): 901–4.

Jones, J. E., et al. "Magnesium Metabolism in Hyperthyroidism and Hypothyroidism." *Journal of Clinical Investigation* 45 (1966): 891–900.

Joshi, H., et al. "Pharmacological Evidences for Antiamnesic Potentials of Phyllanthus amarus in Mice." *African Journal Biomedical Research* 10, no. 2 (2009). doi:10.4314/ajbr.v10i2.50622.

Joyce, J., et al. "The Prognosis of Chronic Fatigue and Chronic Fatigue Syndrome." *Q JM: An International Journal of Medicine* 90 (1997): 223–33.

Kahraman, H., et al. "Gastric Emptying Time in Patients with Primary Hypothyroidism." *European Journal of Gastroenterology & Hepatology* 9, no. 9 (1997): 901–4.

Kapoor, L. D. *CRC Handbook of Ayurvedic Medicinal Plants.* Boca Raton, Fla.: CRC Press, 2000.

Kavitha, C., et al. "Coleus forskohlii: A Comprehensive Review on Morphology, Phytochemistry and Pharmacological Aspects." *Journal of Medicinal Plants Research* 4, no. 4 (2010).

Kilon, F. M., et al. "The Effect of Altered Thyroid Function on the Ultrastructure of the Human Liver." *American Journal of Medicine* 50 (1971): 317–24.

Knudsen, N., et al. "Small Differences in Thyroid Function May Be Important for Body Mass Index and the Occurrence of Obesity in the Population." *Journal of Clinical Endocrinology and Metabolism* 90 (2005): 4019–24.

Kordonouri, O., et al. "Thyroid Autoimmunity in Children and Adolescents with Type 1 Diabetes." *Diabetes Care* 25 (2002): 1346–50.

Kraiem, Z., et al. "Effects of Gamma-Interferon on DR Antigen Expression, Growth, 3,5,3'-Triiodothyronine Secretion, Iodide Uptake and Cyclic Adenosine 3',5'-Monophosphate Accumulation in Cultured Human Thyroid Cells." *Journal of Clinical & Endocrinological Metabolism* 71 (1990): 817–24.

Krassas, G. E., and P. Perros. "Thyroid Disease and Male Reproductive Function." *Journal of Endocrinological Investigation* 26 (2003): 372–80.

Krassas, G. E., K. Poppe, and D. Glinoer. "Thyroid Function and Human Reproductive Health." *Endocrine Reviews* 31 (2010): 702–55.

Krieger, J., and C. Schroeder. "Iron Status and Restless Legs Syndrome." *Sleep Medicine Reviews* 5 (2001): 277–86.

Kvetny, J., et al. "Subclinical Hypothyroidism Is Associated with a Low-Grade Inflammation, Increased Triglyceride Levels and Predicts Cardiovascular Disease in Males Below 50 Years." *Clinical Endocrinology* 61 (2004): 232–38.

Laires, M. J., et al. "Role of Cellular Magnesium in Health and Human Disease." *Frontiers in Bioscience* 9 (2004): 262–76.

Landing, B. H., et al. "Antithyroid Antibody and Chronic Thyroiditis in Diabetes." *Journal of Clinical Endocrinology & Metabolism* 23 (1963): 119–20.

Laurberg, P. "Forskolin Stimulation of Thyroid Secretion of T4 and T3." *Federation of European Biochemical Societies,* 170 (1984): 273–76.

Lavie, P. "Sleep-Wake as a Biological Rhythm." *Annual Review of Psychology* (2001): 277.

Luthra, D. "Ocimum sanctum (Tulsi): A Potent Medicinal Herb." *WebmedCentral Pharmacology* 1, no. 11 (2010): WMC001210. doi:10.9754/journal.wmc.2010.001210.

Maggi, M., et al. "Hormonal Causes of Male Sexual Dysfunctions and Their Management (Hyperprolactinemia, Thyroid Disorders, GH Disorders, and DHEA)." *Journal of Sexual Medicine* 10 (2013): 661–77.

Maheshwari, R., et al. "Herbal Antioxidant: An Emerging Health Protector, " *Journal of Pharmacy Research* 2 (2009): 569–73.

Mason, R. L., et al. "Blood Cholesterol Values in Hyperthyroidism and Hypothyroidism—Their Significance." *New England Journal of Medicine* 203 (1930): 1273–78.

Mazor, M., et al. "Human Preterm Birth Is Associated with Systemic and Local Changes in Progesterone/17B-estradiol Ratios." *American Journal of Obstetrics and Gynecology* 171 (1994): 231–36.

McCaffey, C., and G. A. Quamme. "Effects of Thyroid Status on Renal Calcium and Magnesium Handline." *Canadian Journal of Comparative Medicine* 48 (1984): 51–57.

McDermott, M. T., et al. "Subclinical Hypothyroidism Is Mild Thyroid Failure and Should Be Treated." *Journal of Clinical Endocrinology & Metabolism* 86 (2001): 4585–90.

Meena, A. K., et al. "Plants—Herbal Wealth as a Potential Source of Ayurvedic Drugs." *Asian Journal of Traditional Medicines* 4 (2009).

Meletis, C. D., and W. A. Centrone. "Adrenal Fatigue: Enhancing Quality of Life for Patients with a Functional Disorder." *Alternative & Complementary Therapies* 8 (2002): 267–72.

Messarah, M., et al. "Influence of Thyroid Dysfunction on Liver Lipid Peroxidation and Antioxidant Status in Experimental Rats." *Experimental and Toxicologic Pathology* 62 (2010): 301–10.

Michalopoulou, G., et al. "High Serum Cholesterol Levels in Persons with 'High-Normal' TSH Levels: Should One Extend the Definition of Subclinical Hypothyroidism?" *European Journal of Endocrinology* 138 (1998): 141–45.

Middleton, W. R. "Thyroid Hormones and the Gut." *Gut* 12 (1971): 172–77.

Miller, T. M., and R. B. Layzer. "Muscle Cramps." *Muscle & Nerve* 32 (2005): 431–42.

Mishra, L., et al. "Scientific Basis for the Therapeutic Use of Withania somnifera (Ashwagandha)." *Alternative Medicine Review* 5, no. 4 (2000): 334–46.

Monti, J. M. "Primary and Secondary Insomnia: Prevalence, Causes and Current Therapeutics." *Current Medicinal Chemistry—Central Nervous System Agents* 4 (2004): 119–37.

Mounsey, A. L., and S. W. Reed. "Diagnosing and Treating Hair Loss." *American Family Physician* 80 (2009): 356–62.

Negro, R., et al. "Increased Pregnancy Loss Rate in Thyroid Antibody Negative Women with TSH Levels between 2.5 and 5.0 in the First Trimester of Pregnancy." *Journal of Clinical Endocrinology & Metabolism* 95 (2010): E44–48.

Norris, F. H., and B. J. Fanner. "Hypothyroid Myopathy: Clinical, Electromyographical and Ultrastructural Observations." *Archives of Neurology* 14 (1966): 574–89.

Panda, S. "Changes in Thyroid Hormone Concentrations after Administration of Ashwagandha Root Extract to Adult Male Mice." *Journal of Pharmacy and Pharmacology* 50 (1998): 1065–68.

Panda, S., et al. "Ocimum sanctum Leaf Extract in the Regulation of Thyroid Function in the Male Mouse." *Pharmacological Research* 38 (1998): 107–10.

Pannain, S., and E. Van Cauter. "Modulation of Endocrine Function by Sleep-Wake Homeostasis and Circadian Rhythmicity." *Sleep Medicine Clinics* 2 (2007): 147–59.

Parker, D. C., et al. "Effect of 64-Hour Sleep Deprivation on the Circadian Waveform of Thyrotropin (TSH): Further Evidence of Sleep-Related Inhibition of TSH Release." *Journal of Clinical Endocrinology & Metabolism* 64 (1987): 157–61.

Pereira, J. C., et al. "Imbalance between Thyroid Hormones and the Dopaminergic System Might Be Central to the Pathophysiology of Restless Legs Syndrome: A Hypothesis." *Clinics* 65 (2010): 548–54.

Petajan, J. H. "Pathophysiological Aspects of Human Adjustment to Cold." *Archives of Environmental Health: An International Journal* 17 (1968): 595–98.

Poncin, S., et al. "Oxidative Stress in the Thyroid Gland: From Harmlessness to Hazard Depending on the Iodine Content." *Endocrinology* 149 (2007): 424–33.

Poppe, K., et al. "The Role of Thyroid Autoimmunity in Fertility and Pregnancy." *Nature Clinical Practice: Endocrinology & Metabolism* 4 (2008): 394–405.

Poppe, K., et al. "Thyroid Autoimmunity and Hypothyroidism before and during Pregnancy." *Human Reproduction Update* 9 (2003): 149–61.

Poppe, K., et al. "Thyroid Disease and Female Reproduction." *Clinical Endocrinology* 66 (2007): 309–21.

Prange, A. J., et al. "Effects of Thyrotropin-Releasing hormone in Depression." *Lancet* 300 (1972): 999–1002.

Prummel, M. F., and W. M. Wiersinga. "Thyroid Autoimmunity and Miscarriage." *European Journal of Endocrinology* 150 (2004): 751–55.

Pucci, E., et al. "Thyroid and Lipid Metabolism." *International Journal of Obesity* 24 (2000): S109–12.

Raftogianis, R., et al. "Estrogen Metabolism by Conjugation." *Journal of the National Cancer Institute Monographs* 27 (2000): 113–24.

Rami, B., et al. "Primary Hypothyroidism, Central Diabetes Insipidus and Growth Hormone Deficiency in Multisystem Langerhans Cell Histiocytosis: A Case Report." *Acta Peaediatrica* 87 (1998): 112–14.

Rando, G., and W. Wahli. "Sex Differences in Nuclear Receptor-Regulated Liver Metabolic Pathways." *Biochemica et Biophysica Acta* 3 (2011): 964–73.

Redmond, G. P. "Thyroid Dysfunction and Women's Reproductive Health." *Thyroid* 14 (2004): 5–15.

Reinehr, T. "Obesity and Thyroid Function." *Molecular and Cellular Endocrinology* 316 (2010): 165–71.

Reinehr, T., et al. "Thyroid Hormones and Their Relation to Weight Status." *Hormone Research* 70 (2008): 51–57.

Riddlesberger, M. M., et al. "The Association of Juvenile Hypothyroidism and Cystic Ovaries." *Radiology* 139 (1981): 77–80.

Riley, W. J., et al. "Thyroid Autoimmunity in Insulin-Dependent Diabetes Mellitus: The Case for Routine Screening." *Journal of Pediatrics* 99 (1981): 350–54.

Rizner, T. L., et al. "AKR1C1 and AKR1C3 May Determine Progesterone and Estrogen Ratios in Endometrial Cancer." *Molecular and Cellular Endocrinology* 248 (2006): 126–35.

Rodondi, N., et al. "Subclinical Hypothyroidism and the Risk of Coronary Heart Disease and Mortality." *Journal of the American Medical Association* 304 (2010): 1365–74.

Rosen, R. C. "Correlates of Sexually Related Personal Distress in Women with Low Sexual Desire." *Journal of Sexual Medicine* 6 (2009): 1549–60.

Rox, C. S., et al. "Relations of Thyroid Function to Body Weight." *Archives of Internal Medicine* 1668 (2008): 587–92.

Runahashi, H., et al. "Seaweed Prevents Breast Cancer?" *Cancer Science* 92 (2002): 438–87.

Rupp, J. J. "Hypothyroidism and Diabetes Mellitus." *Diabetes* 4 (1955): 393–97.

Ryuzo, S., and S. Nishiyama. "Alopecia in Hypothyroidism." *Hair Research: Status and Future Aspects; Proceedings of the First International Congress on Hair Research,* Conference Paper, Hamburg, March 13–16, 1979.

Sato, I., et al. "Inhibition of 1251 Organification and Thyroid Hormone Release by Interleukin-1, Tumor Necrosis Factor-Alpha and Interferon-Gamma in Human Thymocytes in Suspension Culture." *Journal of Clinical & Endocrinological Metabolism* 70 (1990): 1735–43.

Savoie, J. C., et al. "Iodine-Induced Thyrotoxicosis in Apparently Normal Thyroid Glands." *Journal of Clinical Endocrinology & Metabolism* 41 (2016): 685–91.

Scanlon, M. F., et al. "Dopaminergic Modulation of Circadian Thyrotropin Rhythm and Thyroid Hormone Levels in Euthyroid Subjects." *Journal of Clinical Endocrinology & Metabolism* 51 (1980): 1251–56.

Selye, Hans. *The Stress of Life.* New York: McGraw-Hill Education, 1978.

Shapiro, J. "Hair Loss in Women." *New England Journal of Medicine* 357 (2007): 1620–30.

Shapiro, J., et al. "Practical Management of Hair Loss." *Canadian Family Physician* 46 (2000): 1469–77.

Sharma, K. "Asparagus racemosus (Shatavari)." *International Journal of Pharmaceutical & Biological Archives* 2 (2011).

Shilo, S., and H. J. Hirsch. "Iodine-Induced Hyperthyroidism in a Patient with a Normal Thyroid Gland." *Postgraduate Medical Journal* 62 (1986): 661–62.

Shu, J., et al. "Ignored Adult Primary Hypothyroidism Presenting Chiefly with Persistent Ovarian Cysts: A Need for Increased Awareness." *Reproductive Biology and Endocrinology* 9 (2011). doi:10.1186/1477-7827-9-119.

Sinaii, N., et al. "High Rates of Autoimmune and Endocrine Disorders, Fibromyalgia, Chronic Fatigue Syndrome and Atopic Diseases among Women with Endometriosis: A Survey Analysis." *Human Reproduction* 17 (2002): 2715–24.

Singh, B. M., et al. "Ovarian Cyst in Juvenile Hypothyroidism." *Archives of Gynecology and Obstetrics* 271 (2005): 263–64.

Singh, S. K., and K. Rajoria. "Evaluation of Vardhamana Pipali, Kanchanar Guggulu and Lekhana Basti in the Management of Hypothyroidism." *Indian Journal of Traditional Knowledge* 14 (2015).

Slok, S., et al. "Plant Profile, Phytochemistry and Pharmacology of Asparagus racemosus (Shatavari)." *Asian Pacific Journal of Tropical Disease* 3 (2013): 242–51.

Smithson, M. J. "Screening for Thyroid Dysfunction in a Community Population of Diabetic Patients." *Diabetic Medicine* 15 (1998): 148–50.

Smyth, P. P. A. "Thyroid Disease and Breast Cancer." *Journal of Endocrinological Investigation* 16 (1993): 396–401.

Stagnaro-Green, A., et al. "Guidelines of the American Thyroid Association for the Diagnosis and Management of Thyroid Disease during Pregnancy and Postpartum." *Thyroid* 21 (2011): 1081–125.

Stagnaro-Green, A., et al. "The Thyroid and Pregnancy: A Novel Risk Factor for Very Preterm Delivery." *Thyroid* 4 (2005): 351–57.

Stagnaro-Green, A., et al. "Thyroid Autoimmunity and the Risk of Miscarriage." *Best Practice & Research: Clinical Endocrinology & Metabolism* 18 (2004): 167–81.

Stanbury, J. B. "Iodine-Induced Hyperthyroidism: Occurrence and Epidemiology." *Thyroid* 8 (1998): 83–100.

Sternbach, H. "Age-Associated Testosterone Decline in Men: Clinical Issues for Psychiatry." *American Journal of Psychiatry* 155 (1998): 1310–18.

Streeten, D. H. P. "Idiopathic Edema: Pathogenesis, Clinical Features, and Treatment." *Metabolism* 27 (1978): 353–83.

Suraj, P., et al. "Shilajit: A Review." *Psychotherapy Research* 21 (2007): 401–5.

Surapaneni, D., et al. "Shilajit Attenuates Behavioral Symptoms of Chronic Fatigue Syndrome by Modulating the Hypothalamic-Pituitary-Adrenal Axis and Mitochondrial Bioenergetics in Rats." *Journal of Ethnopharmacology* 143 (2012): 91–99.

Surks, M. I., et al. "Subclinical Thyroid Disease." *Journal of the American Medical Association* 291 (2004): 228–38.

Takeuchi, K., et al. "A Case of Multiple Ovarian Cysts in a Prepubertal Girl with Severe Hypothyroidism Due to Autoimmune Thyroiditis." *International Journal Gynecological Cancer* 14 (2004): 543–45.

Thangaratinam, S., et al. "Association between Thyroid Autoantibodies and Miscarriage and Preterm Birth." *British Medical Journal* 342 (2011): 2616.

Thompson, W. G., et al. "Functional Bowel Disorders and Functional Abdominal Pain." *Gut* 45 (1999): 1143–47.

Tobin, M. V., et al. "Orocaecal Transit Time in Health and in Thyroid Disease." *Gut* 30 (1989): 26–29.

Tory D. J., et al. "Acute and Delayed Effects of a Single-Dose Injection of Interleukin-6 on Thyroid Function in Healthy Humans." *Metabolism* 47 (1998): 1289–93.

Tribulova, N., et al. "Thyroid Hormones and Cardiac Arrhythmias." *Vascular Pharmacology* 52 (2010): 102–12.

Trokoudes, K. M., et al. "Infertility and Thyroid Disorders." *Current Opinion in Obstetrics and Gynecology* 18 (2006): 446–51.

Tsigos, C., et al. "Hypothalamic-Pituitary-Adrenal Axis, Neuroendocrine Factors and Stress." *Journal of Psychosomatic Research* 53 (2002): 865–71.

Turnbridge, W. M. G., et al. "The Spectrum of Thyroid Disease in a Community: The Whickham Survey." *Clinical Endocrinology* 7 (1977): 481–93.

van Been, N., et al. "Thyroid Hormones Directly Alter Human Hair Follicle Functions." *Journal of Clinical Endocrinology & Metabolism* 93 (2008): 4381–88.

Van den Berghe, G., et al. "Dopamine and the Sick Euthyroid Syndrome in Critical Illness." *Clinical Endocrinology* 41 (1994): 731–37.

Van den Boogaard, E., et al. "Significance of (Sub)clinical Thyroid Dysfunction and Thyroid Autoimmunity before Conception and in Early Pregnancy." *Human Reproduction Update* 17 (2011): 605–19.

Van Sande, J., et al. "Stimulation by Forskolin of the Thyroid Adenylate Cyclase, Cyclic AMP Accumulation and Iodine Metabolism." *Molecular & Cellular Endocrinology* 29 (1983): 109–19.

Vaquero, E., et al. "Mild Thyroid Abnormalities and Recurrent Spontaneous Abortion: Diagnostic and Therapeutical Approach." *American Journal of Reproductive Immunology* 43 (2000): 204–8.

Veronelli, A., et al. "Sexual Dysfunction Is Frequent In Premenopausal Women with Diabetes, Obesity, and Hypothyroidism, and Correlates with Markers of Increased Cardiovascular Risk. A Preliminary Report." *Journal of Sexual Medicine* 6 (2009): 1561–68.

Volzke, H., et al. "Association between Thyroid Function and Gallstone Disease." *World Journal of Gastroenterology* 11, no. 35 (2005): 5530–34.

Vondra, K., et al. "Thyroid Gland Diseases in Adult Patients with Diabetes Mellitus." *Minerva Endocrinologica* 30 (2005): 217–36.

Wajner, S. M. "IL-6 Promotes Nonthyroidal Illness Syndrome by Blocking Thyroxine Activation while Promoting Thyroid Hormone Inactivation in Human Cells." *Journal of Clinical Investigation* 121 (2011): 1834–45.

Wajner, S. M., et al. "Clinical Implications of Altered Thyroid Status in Male Testicular Function." *Arquivos Brasileiros de Endocrinologia e Metabologia* 53, no. 8 (2009): 976–82.

Wassen, F. W., et al. "Effects of Interleukin-1 Beta on Thyrotropin Secretion and Thyroid Hormone Uptake in Cultured Rat Anterior Pituitary Cells." *Endocrinology* 137 (1996): 1591–98.

Weisskopf, A. "Reflux Esophagitis: A Cause of Globus." *Otolaryngology—Head and Neck Surgery* 89, no. 5 (1981): 780–82.

Whiting, D. A. "Chronic Telogen Effluvium: Increased Scalp Hair Shedding in Middle-Aged Women." *Journal of the American Academy of Dermatology* 35 (1996): 899–906.

Whybrow, P. C., et al. "Mental Changes Accompanying Thyroid Gland Dysfunction: A Reappraisal Using Objective Psychological Measurement." *Archives of General Psychiatry* 20 (1969): 48–63.

Wilson, E., et al. "Review of Shilajit Used in Traditional Indian Medicine." *Journal of Ethnopharmacology* 136 (2011): 1–9.

Yun, K., et al. "Effects of Forskolin on the Morphology and Function of the Rat Thyroid Cell Strain." *Journal of Endocrinology* 111 (1986): 397–405.

Ziauddin, M., et al. "Studies on the Immunomodulatory Effects of Ashwagandha." *Journal of Ethnopharmacology* 50 (1996): 69–76.

5. HASHIMOTO'S THYROIDITIS: AUTOIMMUNE DISEASE OF THE THYROID GLAND

Abdei-Rahman, S. Z., et al. "A Multiplex PCR Procedure for Polymorphic Analysis of GSTM1 and GSTT1 Genes in Population Studies." *Cancer Letters* 107 (1996): 229–33.

Abenavoli, L., et al. "Milk Thistle in Liver Diseases: Past, Present, Future." *Phytotherapy Research* 24 (2010): 1423–32.

Abrahamsson, T. R., et al. "Gut Microbiota and Allergy: The Importance of the Pregnancy Period." *Pediatric Research* 77 (2015): 214–19.

Aher, V. D., and A. Wahi. "Pharmacological Study of Tinospora cordifolia as an Immunomodulator." *International Journal of Current Pharmaceutical Research* 2 (2010): 52–54.

Ahmed, A. A., et al. "Gender and Risk of Autoimmune Diseases: Possible Role of Estrogenic Compounds." *Environmental Health Perspectives* 107 (1999): 681–86.

Ait-Beignaoui, A., et al. "Prevention of Gut Leakiness by a Probiotic Treatment Leads to Attenuated HPA Response to an Acute Psychological Stress in Rats." *Psychoneuroendocrinology* 37 (2012): 1885–95.

Al-Asmakh, M., et al. "Gut Microbial Communities Modulating Brain Development and Function." *Journal of Gut Microbes* 3 (2012): 366–73.

Andre, C. "Food Allergy: Objective Diagnosis and Test of Therapeutic Efficacy by Measuring Intestinal Permeability." *Presse Medicine* 15 (1986): 105–8.

Arnson, Y., et al. "Vitamin D and Autoimmunity." *Annals of the Rheumatic Diseases* 66 (2007): 1137–42.

Arora, R. B., et al. "Anti-inflammatory Studies on Curcuma longa (Turmeric)." *Indian Journal of Medical Research* 59 (1971): 1289–95.

Babb, R. R. "Associations between Diseases of the Thyroid and the Liver." *American Journal of Gastroenterology* 79 (1984): 421–23.

Baliga, M. S., et al. "Amla, a Wonder Berry in the Treatment and Prevention of Cancer." *European Journal of Cancer Prevention* 20 (2011): 225–39.

Barile, D., et al. "Human Milk and Related Oligosaccharides as Prebiotics." *Current Opinion in Biotechnology* 24 (2013): 214–19.

Battersby, A. J., and D. L. Gibbons. "The Gut Mucosal Immune System in the Neonatal Period." *Pediatria Allergy and Immunology* 24 (2013): 414–21.

Behrens, R. H., et al. "Factors Affecting the Integrity of the Intestinal Mucosa of Gambian Children." *American Journal of Clinical Nutrition* 45 (1987): 1433–41.

Berti, Irene, et al. "Usefulness of Screening Program for Celiac Disease in Autoimmune Thyroiditis." *Digestive Diseases and Sciences* 45 (2000): 403–6.

Bhandari, P., et al. "Emblica officinalis (Amla): A Review of Potential Therapeutic Applications." *International Journal of Green Pharmacy* 6 (2012): 257–69.

Bhattacharyya, C., and G. Bhattacharyya. "Therapeutic Potential of Tinospora cordifolia: The Magical Herb of Ayurveda." *International Journal of Pharmaceutical & Biological Archives* 4 (2013): 558–84.

Bischoff, S. C. "Gut Health: A New Objective in Medicine?" *Biomedical Central Medicine* 9 (2011): 24.

Bjarnason, I., et al. "Effect of Non-steroidal Anti-inflammatory Drugs on the Human Small Intestine." *Drugs* 1 (1986): 35–41.

Brattstrom, L., et al. "A Common Methylenetetrahydrofolate Reductase Gene Mutation and Longevity." *Atherosclerosis* 141 (1998): 315–19.

Burton, G. W., et al. "Human Plasma and Tissue Alpha-Tocopherol Concentrations in Response to Supplementation with Deuterated Natural and Synthetic Vitamin E." *American Journal of Clinical Nutrition* 67 (1998): 669–84.

Carlson, A. L., et al. "Infant Gut Microbiome Associated with Cognitive Development." *Biological Psychiatry* 83, no. 2 (2017): 148–59.

Cerf-Bensussan, N., and V. Gaboriau-Routhiau. "The Immune System and the Gut Microbiota: Friends or Foes?" *Nature Reviews: Immunology* 10 (2010): 735–44.

Charmkar, N. K., and R. Singh. "Emblica officinalis (Amla): A Wonder Gift of Nature to Humans." *International Journal of Current Microbiology and Applied Sciences* 6 (2017): 4267–80.

Chatterjee, S., et al. "Pesticide Induced Marrow Toxicity and Effects on Marrow Cell Population and on Hematopoietic Stroma." *Experimental and Toxicologic Pathology* 65 (2013): 287–95.

Chattopadhyay, I., et al. "Turmeric and Curcumin: Biological Actions and Medicinal Applications." *Current Science* 87 (2004): 44–50.

Chervonsky, A. V. "Influence of Microbial Environment on Autoimmunity." *Nature Immunology* 11 (2010): 28–35.

Clavel, T., et al. "Deciphering Interactions between the Gut Microbiota and the Immune System via Microbial Cultivation and Minimal Microbiomes." *Immunological Reviews* 279 (2017): 8–22.

Clement, B. "Nutri-Con: The Truth about Vitamins & Supplements." Organic Consumers Association, December 31, 2006. www.organicconsumers.org /news/nutri-con-truth-about-vitamins-supplements.

Cosnes, J., et al. "Incidence of Autoimmune Diseases in Celiac Disease." *Clinical Gastroenterology and Hepatology* 6 (2008): 753–58.

Crissinger, K. D., et al. "Pathophysiology of Gastrointestinal Mucosal Permeability." *Journal of Internal Medicine Supplement* 732 (1990): 145–54.

Deloughery, T. G., et al. "Common Mutation in Methylenetetrahydrofolate Reductase." *Circulation* 94 (1996): 3074–78.

Deluca, H. F., and M. T. Cantorna. "Vitamin D: Its Role and Uses in Immunology." *Federation of American Societies for Experimental Biology (FASEB) Journal* 15 (2001): 2579–85.

Desai, V. R., et al. "An Immunomodulator from Tinospora cordifolia with Antioxidant Activity in Cell-Free Systems." *Journal of Chemical Sciences* 114 (2002): 713–19.

Doe, W. F. "An Overview of Intestinal Immunity and Malabsorption." *American Journal of Medicine* 67 (1979): 1077–84.

Elfstrom, P., et al. "Risk of Thyroid Disease in Individuals with Celiac Disease." *Journal of Clinical Endocrinology & Metabolism* 93 (2008): 3915–21.

Fahey, J. W. "Moringa oleifera: A Review of the Medicinal Evidence for Its Nutritional, Therapeutic and Prophylactic Properties, Part 1." *Trees for Life Journal* 1 (2005): 5.

Fakurazi, S., et al. "Moringa oleifera Prevents Acetaminophen Induced Liver Injury through Restoration of Glutathione Level." *Food and Chemical Toxicology* 46 (2008): 2611–15.

Fasano, A. "Leaky Gut and Autoimmune Diseases." *Clinical Reviews in Allergy & Immunology* 42 (2012): 71–78.

Fernandez, L., et al. "The Human Milk Microbiota." *Pharmacological Research 69 (2013): 1–10.*

Ferreira, P. M. P., et al. "Moringa oleifera: Bioactive Compounds and Nutritional Potential." *Review of Nutrition* 21 (2008): 431–37.

Francino, M. P. "Early Development of the Gut Microbiota and Immune Health." *Pathogens* 3 (2014): 769–90.

Galland, L., and S. Barrie. "Intestinal Dysbiosis and the Causes of Disease." *Journal for the Advancement of Medicine* 6 (1993): 67–82.

Gautam, R., et al. "Folk Medicinal Uses of Plants from Kusmi Forest, Uttar Pradesh, Gorakhpur, India." *International Journal of Current Microbiology and Applied Sciences* 4 (2014): 343–51.

Ghaisas, S., et al. "Gut Microbiome in Health and Disease." *Pharmacology & Therapeutics* 158 (2016): 52–62.

Ghildiyal, J. C., et al. "Indigenous Uses of Plants in Different Women Ailments in Garhwal Region." *Indian Journal of Pharmaceutical and Biological Research* 2 (2014): 39–44.

Gorbach, S. L. "Estrogens, Breast Cancer and Intestinal Flora." *Reviews of Infectious Diseases* 6 (1984): S85–90.

Gritz, E. C., and V. Bhandari. "The Human Neonatal Gut Microbiome." *Frontiers in Pediatrics* 3 (2015): 60.

Gudmundsdottir, K., et al. "GSTM1 GSTT1 and GSTP1 Genotypes in Relation to Breast Cancer Risk and Frequency of Mutations in the p53 Gene." *Cancer Epidemiology, Biomarkers & Prevention* 10 (2001): 1169–73.

Group, E. "The Differences between Synthetic and Natural Vitamins." *Global Healing,* January 2009. Last updated June 16, 2017.

Guest, I., et al. "Drugs Toxic to the Bone Marrow That Target the Stromal Cells." *Immunopharmacology* 46 (2000): 103–12.

Hardy, H., et al. "Probiotics, Prebiotics and Immunomodulation of Gut Mucosal Defences: Homeostasis and Immunopathology." *Nutrients* 5 (2013): 1869–912.

Hawrelak, J. "Probiotics, Prebiotics and Synbiotics." *Journal of Complementary Medicine* 6 (2007): 28–35.

Hawrelak, J. A. "The Causes of Intestinal Dysbiosis." *Alternative Medicine Review* 9 (2004): 180–97.

Heijmans, B. T., et al. "Mortality Risk in Men Is Associated with a Common Mutation in the Methylenetetrahydrofolate Reductase Gene (MTHFR)." *European Journal of Human Genetics* 7 (1999): 197–204.

Hooper, L. V., et al. "Interactions between the Microbiota and the Immune System." *Science* 336 (20012): 1268–73.

Husain, S., et al. "Hepatoprotective, Anticancer and Antiviral Effects of Bhumi Amla in Unani Medicine." *Journal of Medicinal Plants Studies* 3 (2015): 1–3.

Inoue, Y., and N. Shimojo. "Microbiome/Microbiota and Allergies." *Seminars in Immunopathology* 37 (2015): 56–64.

Jackson, P. G., et al. "Intestinal Permeability in Patients with Eczema and Food Allergy." *Lancet* 1 (1981): 1285–86.

Jalonen, T. "Identical Intestinal Permeability Changes in Children with Different Clinical Manifestations of Cow's Milk Allergy." *Journal of Allergy & Clinical Immunology* 88 (1991): 737–42.

Jeon, Y. J., et al. "Effects of Beta-carotene Supplements on Cancer Prevention." *Nutrition and Cancer* 63 (2011): 1196–207.

Jernberg, C., et al. "Long-Term Impacts of Antibiotic Exposure on the Human Intestinal Microbiota." *Microbiology* 156 (2010): 3216–23.

Jeurink, P. V., et al. "Human Milk: A Source of More Life Than We Imagine." *Beneficial Microbes* 4 (2012): 17–30.

Jeyachandran, R., et al. "Antibacterial Activity of Stem Extracts of Tinospora cordifolia." *Ancient Science of Life* 23 (2003): 40–43.

Kapli, A., et al. "Immunopotentiating Compounds from Tinospora cordifolia." *Journal of Ethnopharmacology* 58 (1997): 89–95.

Kelly, P. "Nutrition, Intestinal Defence and the Microbiome." *Proceedings of the Nutrition Society* 69 (2010): 261–68.

Kerr, C. A., et al. "Early Life Events Influence Whole-of-Life Metabolic Health via Gut Microflora and Gut Permeability." *Critical Reviews in Microbiology* 41 (2015): 326–40.

Khopde, S. M., et al. "Characterizing the Antioxidant Activity of Amla Extract." *Current Science* 81 (2001): 185–90.

Khosla, S., and S. Sharma. "A Short Description on Pharmacogenetic Properties of Emblica officinalis." *ScopeMed* 2 (2012): 187–93.

Kim, B. "Synthetic vs. Natural Vitamins." Dr. Ben Kim's blog, posted October 3, 2004.

Klein, S. L., et al. "Sex-Based Difference in Immune Function and Responses to Vaccination." *Transactions of the Royal Society of Tropical Medicine and Hygiene* 109 (2015): 9–15.

Kong, J., et al. "Novel Role of the Vitamin D Receptor in Maintaining the Integrity of the Intestinal Mucosal Barrier." *American Journal of Physiology, Gastrointestinal and Liver* 294 (2007): G208–16.

Konkel, L. "The Environment Within: Exploring the Role of the Gut Microbiome in Health and Disease." *Environmental Health Perspectives* 121 (2013): A276–81.

Kosower, N. S., et al. "The Glutathione Status of Cells." *International Review of Cytology* 54 (1978): 109–60.

Kramer, K. "Stomach Disorders." *Journal of Complementary Medicine* 2 (2003): 24–28.

Kuftan, R., et al. "Potential Anticancer Activity of Turmeric (Curcuma longa)." *Cancer Letters* 29 (1985): 197–202.

Kumar, N., et al. "Leafy Drugs from Tehsil Joginder Nagar, District Mandi, Himachal Pradesh, India." *Research in Pharmacy* 4 (2014).

Kumar, S., et al. "Free and Bound Phenolic Antioxidants in Amla (Emblica officinalis) and Turmeric (Curcuma longa)." *Journal of Food Composition and Analysis* 19 (2006): 446–52.

Kumari, M. "Evaluation of Methanolic Extracts of In Vitro Grown Tinospora cordifolia for Antibacterial Activities." *Asian Journal of Pharmaceutical and Clinical Research* 5 (2012): 172–75.

Kussmann, M., and P. J. Van Bladeren. "The Extended Nutrigenomics—Understanding the Interplay between the Genomes of Food, Gut Microbes, and Human Host." *Frontiers in Genetics* 2 (2011): 21.

Kuttan, R., and K. B. Harikumar. *Phyllanthus Species.* Boca Raton, Fla.: CRC Press, 2012.

Land, C. A., et al. "Low Blood Glutathione Levels in Healthy Aging Adults." *Journal of Laboratory and Clinical Medicine* 120 (1992): 720–25.

Lang, K. S., et al. "The Role of the Innate Immune Response in Autoimmune Disease." *Journal of Autoimmunity* 29 (2007): 206–12.

LaTuga, M. S., et al. "A Review of the Source and Function of Microbiota in Breast Milk." *Seminars in Reproductive Medicine* 32 (2014): 68–73.

Le Bousse-Kerdiles, M., et al. "Cellular and Molecular Mechanisms Underlying Bone Marrow and Liver Fibrosis." *European Cytokine Network* 19 (2008): 69–80.

Lobo, V., et al. "Free Radicals, Antioxidants and Functional Foods." *Pharmacognosy Reviews* 4 (2010): 118–26.

Maes, M., et al. "The Gut-Brain Barrier in Major Depression: Intestinal Mucosal Dysfunction with an Increased Translocation of LPS from Gram Negative Enterobacteria (Leaky Gut) Plays a Role in the Inflammatory Pathophysiology of Depression." *Neuroendocrinology Letters* 29 (2008): 117–24.

Maes, M., et al. "Normalization of Leaky Gut in Chronic Fatigue Syndrome (CFS) Is Accompanied by a Clinical Improvement." *Neuroendocrinology Letters* 29 (2008): 101–9.

Maggini, S., et al. "Selected Vitamins and Trace Elements Support Immune Function by Strengthening Epithelial Barriers and Cellular and Humoral Immune Responses." *British Journal of Nutrition* 98 (2007): 529–35.

Makkar, H. P. S., and K. Becker. "Nutrients and Antiquity Factors in Different Morphological Parts of the Moringa oleifera Tree." *Journal of Agricultural Science* 128 (1997): 311–22.

Malmuthuge, N., et al. "Heat-Treated Colostrum Feeding Promotes Beneficial Bacteria Colonization in the Small Intestine of Neonatal Calves." *Journal of Dairy Science* 98 (2015): 8044–53.

Marques, T. M., et al. "Gut Microbiota Modulation and Implications for Host Health." *Innovative Food Science & Emerging Technologies* 22 (2014): 239–47.

Marrack, P., et al. "Autoimmune Disease: Why and Where It Occurs." *Nature Medicine* 7 (2001): 899.

Matsushita, S., et al. "The Frequency of the Methylenetetrahydrofolate Reductase-Gene Mutation Varies with Age in the Normal Population." *American Journal of Human Genetics* 6 (1997): 1459–60.

Matthew, S., et al. "Immunomodulatory and Anti-Tumour Activities of Tinospora cordifolia." *Fitoterapia* 70 (1999): 35–43.

McGuire, M. K., et al. "Got Bacteria? The Astounding, yet Not-So-Surprising, Microbiome of Human Milk." *Current Opinion in Biotechnology* 44 (2017): 63–68.

Meister, A., and M. E. Anderson. "Glutathione." *Annual Review of Biochemistry* 52 (1983): 711–60.

Mishra, S., and K. Palanivelu. "The Effect of Curcumin (Turmeric) on Alzheimer's Disease: An Overview." *Annals of Indian Academy of Neurology* 11 (2008): 13–19.

Mitchell, J. R., et al. "Acetaminophen-Induced Hepatic Necrosis. Protective Role of Glutathione." *Journal of Pharmacology and Experimental Therapeutics* 187 (1973): 211–17.

Molina, V., and Y. Shoenfeld. "Infection, Vaccines and Other Environmental Triggers of Autoimmunity." *Journal of Autoimmunity* 38 (2005): 235–45.

Mori, K., et al. "Does the Gut Microbiota Trigger Hashimoto's Thyroiditis?" *Discovery Medicine* 14, no. 78 (2012): 321–26.

Moyo, B., et al. "Nutritional Characterization of Moringa oleifera Leaves." *African Journal of Biotechnology* 10 (2011): 12925–33.

Mueller, N. T., et al. "The Infant Microbiome Development: Mom Matters." *Trends in Molecular Medicine* 21, no. 2 (2015): 109–17.

Munblit, D., et al. "Exposures Influencing Total IgA Level in Colostrum." *Journal of Developmental Origins of Health and Disease* 7 (2016): 61–67.

Mursu, J., et al. "Dietary Supplements and Mortality Rate in Older Women: The Iowa Women's Health Study." *Archives of Internal Medicine* 171 (2011): 1625–33.

Narendra, K., et al. "Phyllanthus niruri: A Review on Its Ethno Botanical, Phytochemical and Pharmacological Profile." *Journal of Pharmacy Research* 5 (2012): 4681–91.

Neu, J. "The Developing Intestinal Microbiome: Probiotics and Prebiotics." *Nature* 457 (2009): 480–84.

Neuhouser, M. L., et al. "Multivitamin Use and Risk of Cancer and Cardiovascular Disease in the Women's Health Initiative Cohorts." *Archives of Internal Medicine* 169 (2008): 294–304.

Newburg, D. S., and Y. He. "Neonatal Gut Microbiota and Human Milk Glycans Cooperate to Attenuate Infection and Inflammation." *Clinical Obstetrics and Gynecology* 58 (2015): 814–26.

Nimse, S. B., and D. Pal. "Free Radicals, Natural Antioxidants, and Their Reaction Mechanisms." *Royal Society of Chemistry* 5 (2015): 27986–8006.

O'Callaghan, T. F., et al. "The Gut Microbiome as a Virtual Endocrine Organ with Implications for Farm and Domestic Animal Endocrinology." *Domestic Animal Endocrinology* 56 (2016): S44–55.

Odenwald, M. A., et al. "Intestinal Permeability Defects: Is It Time to Treat?" *Clinical Gastroenterology and Hepatology* 11 (2013): 1075–83.

Ohteki, T., et al. "Liver Is a Possible Site for the Proliferation of Abnormal CD3+4-8-Double-Negative Lymphocytes in Autoimmune MRS-lpr/lpr Mice." *Journal of Experimental Medicine* 172 (1990): 7.

O'Mahony, S. M., et al. "Early-Life Adversity and Brain Development: Is the Microbiome a Missing Piece of the Puzzle?" *Neuroscience* 342 (2017): 37–54.

O'Sullivan, A., et al. "Early Diet Impacts Infant Rhesus Gut Microbiome, Immunity and Metabolism." *Journal of Proteome Research* 12 (2013): 2833–45.

Paganelli, R., et al. "Intestinal Permeability in Irritable Bowel Syndrome: Effect of Diet and Sodium Cromoglycate Administration." *Pediatric Gastroenterology & Nutrition* 11 (1990): 72–77.

Pandit, N. "Guduchi: The Amrit of Ayurveda." California College of Ayurveda, 2016. www.ayurvedacollege.com/articles/students/Guduchi.

Parks, S. Y., et al. "Multivitamin Use and the Risk of Mortality and Cancer

Incidence: The Multiethnic Cohort Study." *American Journal of Epidemiology* 173 (2011): 906–14.

Pendse, V. K., et al. "Anti-Inflammatory, Immunosuppressive and Some Related Pharmacological Actions of the Water Extract of Tinospora cordifolia." *Indian Journal of Pharmacology* 9 (1977): 221–24.

Perez-Cobas, A. E., et al. "Gut Microbiota Disturbance during Antibiotic Therapy." *Gut* 62 (2013): 1591–601.

Rautave, S. "Early Microbial Contact, the Breast Milk Microbiome and Child Health." *Journal of Developmental Origins of Health and Disease* 7 (2016): 5–14.

Razis, A., et al. "Health Benefits of Moringa oleifera." *Asian Pacific Journal of Cancer Prevention* 15 (2014): 8571–76.

Rebbeck, T. R. "Molecular Epidemiology of the Human Glutathione S-transferase Genotypes GSTM1 and GSTT1 in Cancer Susceptibility." *Cancer Epidemiology, Biomarkers & Prevention* 6 (1997): 733–43.

Reid, I. R. "Effects of Vitamin D Supplements on Bone Mineral Density." *Lancet* 383 (2014): 146–55.

Rooney, P. J., and R. T. Jenkins. "Nonsteroidal Anti-Inflammatory Drugs (NSAIDs) and the Bowel Mucosa." *Clinical Rheumatology* 8 (1990): 328–29.

Rosana, B., et al. "Should the Human Microbiome Be Considered When Developing Vaccines?" *PLoS Pathogens* 6 (2010). doi:10.1371/journal.ppat.1001190.

Saha, S., and S. Ghosh. "Tinospora cordifolia: One Plant, Many Roles." *Ancient Science of Life* 31 (2012): 151–59.

Sanz, Y. "Gut Microbiota and Probiotics in Maternal and Infant Health." *American Journal of Clinical Nutrition* 94 (2011): 2000S–5S.

Sathyabama, S., et al. "Friendly Pathogens: Prevent or Provoke Autoimmunity." *Critical Reviews in Microbiology* 40 (2014): 273–80.

Saul, A. "What Is the Difference Between Natural and Synthetic Vitamins?" DoctorYourself.Com. Accessed September 2018.

Seki, E., and B. Schnabl. "Role of Innate Immunity and the Microbiota in Liver Fibrosis." *Journal of Physiology* 590 (2012): 447–58.

Sekirov, I., et al. "Antibiotic-Induced Perturbations of the Intestinal Microbiota Alter Host Susceptibility to Enteric Infection." *Infection and Immunity* 76 (2008): 4726–36.

Sela, D. A., et al. "Nursing Our Microbiota: Molecular Linkages between Bifidobacteria and Milk Oligosaccharides." *Trends in Microbiology* 18, no. 7 (2010): 298–307.

Selvam, R., et al. "The Antioxidant Activity of Turmeric (Curcuma longa)." *Journal of Ethnopharmacology* 47 (1999): 59-67.

Sharma, H. "Leaky Gut Syndrome, Dysbiosis, Ama, Free Radicals and Natural Antioxidants." *Ayu Journal* 30 (2009): 88–105.

Sharma, U., et al. "Immunomodulatory Active Compounds from Tinospora cordifolia." *Journal of Ethnopharmacology* 141 (2012): 918–26.

Sharma, V., and D. Pandey. "Protective Role of Tinospora cordifolia against Lead-Induced Hepatotoxicity." *Toxicology International* 17 (2010): 12–17.

Sherman, M. P., et al. "Gut Microbiota, the Immune System, and Diet Influence the Neonatal Gut-Brain Axis." *Pediatric Research* 77 (2015): 127–35.

Sherwin, E., et al. "A Gut (Microbiome) Feeling about the Brain." *Current Opinion in Gastroenterology* 32 (2016): 96–102.

Siddhuraju, P., and K. Becker. "Antioxidant Properties of Various Solvent Extracts of Total Phenolic Constituents from Three Different Agroclimatic Origins of Drumstick Tree (Moringa oleifera) Leaves." *Asian Pacific Journal of Cancer Prevention* 15 (2014): 2144–55.

Sies, H. "Glutathione and Its Role in Cellular Functions." *Free Radical Biology and Medicine* 27 (1999): 916–21.

Singh, N., et al. "Immunomodulatory and Antitumor Actions of Medicinal Plant Tinospora cordifolia Are Mediated through Activation of Tumor-Associated Macrophages." *Immunopharmacology and Immunotoxicology* 26 (2004): 145–62.

Singh, S. S., et al. "Chemistry and Medicinal Properties of Tinospora cordifolia (Guduchi)." *Indian Journal of Pharmacology* 35 (2003): 83–91.

Sun, J. "Vitamin D and Mucosal Immune Function." *Current Opinion in Gastroenterology* 26 (2010): 591–95.

Sunanda, S. N., et al. "Antiallergic Properties of Tinospora cordifolia in Animal Models." *Indian Journal of Pharmacology* 18 (1986): 250–52.

Sutherland, D. B., et al. "IgA Synthesis: A Form of Functional Immune Adaptation Extending beyond Gut." *Current Opinion in Immunology* 24 (2012): 261–68.

Theodoratou, E., et al. "Vitamin D and Multiple Health Outcomes." *British Medical Journal* 348 (2014).

Thiel, R. J. "Natural Vitamins May Be Superior to Synthetic Ones." *Medical Hypotheses* 55 (2000): 461–69.

Tlaskalova-Hogenova, H., et al. "Commensal Bacteria (Normal Microflora), Mucosal Immunity and Chronic Inflammatory and Autoimmune Diseases." *Immunology Letters* 93 (2004): 97–108.

Tlaskalova-Hogenova, H., et al. "The Role of Gut Microbiota and the Mucosal Barrier in the Pathogenesis of Inflammatory and Autoimmune Diseases and Cancer." *Cellular and Molecular Immunology* 8 (2011): 110–20.

Tuzcu, A., et al. "Subclinical Hypothyroidism May Be Associated with Elevated High-Sensitive C-Reactive Protein (Low Grade Inflammation) and Fasting Hyperinsulinemia." *Endocrine Journal* 52 (2005): 89–94.

Uetrecht, J., and D. J. Naisbitt. "Idiosyncratic Adverse Drug Reactions." *Pharmacological Reviews* 65 (2013): 779–808.

Underwood, M. A., et al. "Bifidobacterium longum Subspecies infantis: Champion Colonizer of the Infant Gut." *Pediatria Research* 77 (2015): 229–35.

Vangay, P., et al. "Antibiotics, Pediatric Dysbiosis and Disease." *Cell Host & Microbe* 17 (2015): 553–64.

Velasquez-Manoff, M. "Gut Microbiome: The Peacekeepers." *Nature* 518, no. 7540 (2015): S3–11.

Verma, A. R., et al. "In Vitro and In Vivo Antioxidant Properties of Different Fractions of Moringa oleifera Leaves." *Food and Chemical Toxicology* 47 (2009): 2196–201.

Verma, Sonia, and Reena Hooda. "Microwave Assisted Extraction of Phyllanthus amarus." *Journal of Pharmacognosy and Phytochemistry* 4, no. 1 (2016): 66–77.

Voreades, N., et al. "Diet and the Development of the Human Intestinal Microbiome." *Frontiers in Microbiology* 5 (2014): 494.

Walker, M. "Formula Supplementation of the Breastfed Infant: Assault on the Gut Microbiome." *Clinical Lactation* 5 (2014): 128–32.

Wang, H., et al. "Total Antioxidant Capacity of Fruits." *Journal of Agricultural and Food Chemistry* 44 (1996): 701–5.

Wang, L., et al. "Effects of Chromium on Mouse Oocyte Apoptosis and DNA Damage." *Journal of Shanghai Jiaotong University—Agricultural Science* 27 (2009): 561–65.

Watkins, M. L., et al. "Multivitamin Use and Mortality in a Large Prospective Study." *American Journal of Epidemiology* 152 (2000): 149–62.

Weetman, A. P. "Autoimmune Thyroid Disease." *Autoimmunity* 37 (2009): 337–40.

Wu, G., et al. "Glutathione Metabolism and Its Implications for Health." *Journal of Nutrition* 134 (2004): 489–92.

Yadav, V., et al. "Amla—Medicinal Food and Pharmacological Activity." *International Journal of Pharmaceutical and Chemical Sciences* 3 (2014): 616–19.

Yang, I., et al. "The Infant Microbiome: Implications for Infant Health and Neurocognitive Development." *Nursing Research* 65 (2016): 76–88.

6. GALLBLADDER FUNCTION AND THE THYROID GLAND

Akiba, Y., et al. "Acid-Sensing Pathways of Rat Duodenum." *American Journal of Physiology: Gastrointestinal & Liver* 277 (1999): G268–74.

Arnaud, S. B., et al. "25-hydroxyvitamin D3: Evidence of an Enterohepatic Circulation in Man." *Proceedings of the Society for Experimental Biology and Medicine* 149, no. 2 (1975): 570–72.

Arnett, T. "Regulation of Bone Cell Function by Acid-Base Balance." *Proceedings of the Nutrition Society* 62 (2003): 511–20.

Austin, A. "A Review on Indian Sarsaparilla, Hemidesmus indicus." *Journal of Biological Sciences* 8 (2008): 1–12.

Baheti, J. R., et al. "Hepatoprotective Activity of Hemidesmus indicus R. Br. in Rats." *Indian Journal of Experimental Biology* 44 (2006): 399–402.

Baklanova, V. F., et al. "Effect of Cholosas, Magnesium Sulfate, and Sorbitol on the Motor Function of the Gallbladder in Children." *Pediatriia* 3 (1976): 50–1.

Baliga, M. S., et al. "Use of the Ayurvedic Drug Triphala in Medical Conditions Afflicting Older Adults." *Academic Press* (2015): 135–42.

Barbara, L., et al., eds. *Bile Acids in Gastroenterology: Proceedings of an International Symposium Held at Cortina d'Ampezzo, Italy, 17–20th March 1982.* Boston: MTP Press, 1983.

Behar, J., and P. Biancani. "Effect of Cholecystokinin and the Octapeptide of Cholecystokinin on the Feline Sphincter of Oddi and Gallbladder." *Journal of Clinical Investigation* 66 (1980): 1231–39.

Beil, U., et al. "Effects of Interruption of the Enterohepatic Circulation of Bile Acids on the Transport of Very Low Density-Lipoprotein Triglycerides." *Metabolism* 31 (1982): 438–44.

Bern, A., and W. T. Cooke. "Intraluminal pH of Duodenum and Jejunum in Fasting Subjects with Normal and Abnormal Gastric or Pancreatic Function." *Scandinavian Journal of Gastroenterology* 6 (1971): 313–17.

Buclin, T., et al. "Diet Acids and Alkalis Influence Calcium Retention in Bone." *Osteoporosis International* 12 (2001): 493–99.

Buhman, K. K., et al. "Dietary Psyllium Increases Fecal Bile Acid Excretion, Total Steroid Excretion and Bile Acid Biosynthesis in Rats." *Journal of Nutrition* 128 (1998): 1199–203.

Byers, S. G., and M. Friedman. "Production and Excretion of Cholesterol in Mammals. VII. Biliary Cholesterol: Increment and Indicator of Hepatic Synthesis of Cholesterol." *American Journal of Physiology* 168 (1952): 297–302.

Cahan, M. A., et al. "Proton Pump Inhibitors Reduce Gallbladder Function." *Surgical Endoscopy and Other Interventional Techniques* 20 (2006): 1364–67.

Chey, W. D., et al. "A Randomized Placebo-Controlled Phase IIb Trial of A3309, a Bile Acid Transporter Inhibitor, for Chronic Idiopathic Constipation." *American Journal of Gastroenterology* 106 (2011): 1803–12.

Ciobanu, L., and D. L. Dumitrascu. "Gastrointestinal Motility Disorders in Endocrine Diseases." *Polskie Archiwum Medycyny Wewnetrznej* 121 (2011): 129–36.

Corradini, S. G., et al. "Impaired Human Gallbladder Lipid Absorption in Cholesterol Gallstone Disease and Its Effect on Cholesterol Solubility in Bile." *Gastroenterology* 118 (2000): 912–20.

Daher, R., et al. "Consequences of Dysthyroidism on the Digestive Tract and Viscera." *World Journal of Gastroenterology* 15 (2009): 2834–38.

Das, S. "The Bioactive and Therapeutic Potential of Hemidesmus indicus R. Br. (Indian Sarsaparilla) Root." *Phytotherapy Research* 27 (2013): 791–801.

Dietschy, J. M., et al. "Studies on the mechanisms of Intestinal Transport." *Journal of Clinical Investigation* 45 (1966): 832–46.

Dowling, R. H., et al. "Experimental Model for the Study of Enterohepatic Circulation of Bile in Rhesus Monkeys." *Journal of Laboratory and Clinical Medicine* 72 (1968): 169–76.

Dressman, J. B., et al. "Upper Gastrointestinal (GI) pH in Young, Healthy Men and Women." *Pharmaceutical Research* 7 (1990): 756–61.

Eid, F. A., et al. "Hypolipidemic Effect of Triphala (Terminalia chebula, Terminalia belerica and Emblica officinalis) on Female Albino Rats." *Egyptian Journal of Hospital Medicine* 43 (2011): 226–40.

Eyssen, H. "Role of the Gut Microflora in Metabolism of Lipids and Sterols." *Proceedings of the Nutrition Society* 32 (1973): 59–63.

Fallingborg, J. "Intraluminal pH of the Human Gastrointestinal Tract." *Danish Medical Bulletin* 46 (1999): 183–96.

Fiemstrom, G., and E. Kivilaakso. "Demonstration of a pH Gradient at the Luminal Surface of Rat Duodenum In Vivo and Its Dependence on Mucosal Alkaline Secretion." *Gastroenterology* 84 (1983): 787–94.

Forker, E. L. "The Effect of Estrogen on Bile Formation in the Rat." *Journal of Clinical Investigation* 48 (1969): 654–63.

Frawley, David, and Vasant Lad. *The Yoga of Herbs.* Twin Lakes, Wisc.: Lotus Press, 1986.

Fuchs, M. "III. Regulation of Bile Acid Synthesis: Past Progress and Future Challenges." *American Journal of Physiology: Gastrointestinal & Liver* 284 (2003): G551–57.

Gerbstadt, Christine. *Doctor's Detox Diet.* Sarasota, Fla.: Nutronics, 2012.

Grundy, S. M., E. H. Ahrens, and G. Salen. "Interruption of the Enterohepatic Circulation of Bile Acids in Man: Comparative Effects of Cholestyramine and Ileal Exclusion on Cholesterol Metabolism." *Journal of Laboratory and Clinical Medicine* 78, no. 1 (1971): 94–121.

Grundy, S. M., and S. C. Kaiser. "Highlights of the Meeting on Prevention of Gallstones." *Hepatology* 7 (1987): 946–51.

Gumucio, J. J., et al. "Studies on the Mechanisms of the Ethynylestradiol Impairment of Bile Flow and Bile Salt Excretion in the Rat." *Gastroenterology* 61 (1971): 339–44.

Gunay, A., et al. "Gallbladder and Gastric Motility in Patients with Idiopathic Slow-Transit Constipation." *Southern Medical Journal* (2004): 124.

Hellstrom, P. M. "Role of Bile in Regulation of Gut Motility." *Journal of Internal Medicine* 237 (1995): 395–402.

Hofmann, A. F. "The Continuing Importance of Bile Acids in Liver and Intestinal Disease." *Archives of Internal Medicine* 159 (1999): 2647–58.

Hofmann, A. F. "Enterohepatic Circulation of Bile Acids." *Comprehensive Physiology.* January 1, 2011.

Hofmann, A. F., and L. Eckmann. "How Bile Acids Confer Gut Mucosal Protection against Bacteria." *Proceedings of the National Academy of Sciences* 103 (2017): 4333–34.

Hofmann, Alan F., et al. "Altered Bile Acid Metabolism in Childhood Functional Constipation: Inactivation of Secretory Bile Acids by Sulfation in a Subset of Patients." *Journal of Pediatric Gastroenterology & Nutrition* 47 (2008): 598–606.

Holzbach, R. T., et al. "The Effect of Pregnancy on Lipid Composition of Guinea Pig Gallbladder Bile." *Gastroenterology* 60 (1971): 288–93.

Hurd, K. R. "Gallbladder Disease." Karen R. Hurd Nutritional Practice, LLC, www.karenhurd.com/gallbladder-disease.html. Updated June 16, 2014.

Imamoglu, K., et al. "Production of Gallstones by Prolonged Administration of Progesterone and Estradiol in Rabbits." *Surgical Forum* 10 (1960): 246–49.

Inkinen, J., et al. "Direct Effect of Thyroxine on Pig Sphincter of Oddi Contractility." *Digestive Diseases and Sciences* 46 (2001): 182–86.

Isaksson, B. "On the Dissolving Power of Lecithin and Bile Salts for Cholesterol in Human Bladder Bile." *Acta Societatis Medicorum Upsaliensis* 59 (1954): 296–306.

Kamboj, V. P. "Herbal Medicine." *Current Science* 78 (2000): 35–39.

Kazutomo, I., et al. "Correlation between Gallbladder Size and Release of Cholecystokinin After Oral Magnesium Sulfate in Man." *Annals of Surgery* 197 (1983): 412–15.

Kerckhoffs, D. A., et al. "Cholesterol-Lowering Effect of Beta-glucan from Oat Bran in Mildly Hypercholesterolemic Subjects May Decrease When Beta-glucan Is Incorporated into Bread and Cookies." *American Journal of Clinical Nutrition* 78 (2003): 221–27.

Klaassen, C. D., and J. B. Watkins. "Mechanisms of Bile Formation, Hepatic Uptake and Biliary Excretion." *Pharmacological Reviews* 36 (1984): 1–67.

Kulpers, F., et al. "Enterohepatic Circulation in the Rat." *Gastroenterology* 88 (1985): 403–11.

Lad, Vasant. *Secrets of the Pulse: The Ancient Art of Ayurvedic Pulse Diagnosis.* Albuquerque, N.Mex.: Ayurvedic Press, 1996.

Laukkarinen, J., et al. "Bile Flow to the Duodenum Is Reduced in Hypothyreosis and Enhanced in Hyperthyreosis." *Neurogastroenterology & Motility* 14 (2002): 183–88.

Laukkarinen, J., et al. "Increased Prevalence of Subclinical Hypothyroidism in Common Bile Duct Stone Patients." *Journal of Clinical Endocrinology & Metabolism* 92 (2007): 42260–64.

Laukkarinen, J., et al. "Is Bile Flow Reduced in Patients with Hypothyroidism?" *Surgery* 133 (2003): 288–93.

Layden, T. J., and J. L. Boyer. "The Effect of Thyroid Hormone on Bile Salt-Independent Bile Flow and Na+, K+ -ATPase Activity in Liver Plasma Membranes Enriched in Bile Canaliculi." *Journal of Clinical Investigation* 57 (1976): 1009–18.

Leontowicz, M. "Apple and Pear Peel and Pulp and Their Influence on Plasma Lipids and Antioxidant Potentials in Rats Fed Cholesterol-Containing Diets." *Journal of Agriculture & Food Chemistry* 10 (2003): 5780–85.

Lorenzo, Y., et al. "Hypotonia of the Gallbladder of Myxedematous Origin." *Journal of Clinical Endocrinology & Metabolism* 17 (1957): 133–42.

Lynn, J., et al. "Effects of Estrogen upon Bile: Implications with Respect to Gallstone Formation." *Annals of Surgery* 178 (1973): 514–24.

Malagelada, J. R., et al. "Panaceatic, Gallbladder, and Intestinal Responses to Intraluminal Magnesium Salts in Man." *American Journal of Digestive Diseases* 23 (1978): 481–85.

Maritz, F. J. "Efficacy and Danger of Statin Therapy." *Cardiovascular Journal of South Africa* 13 (2002): 200–3.

Moghadasian, M. H., and J. J. Frohlich. "Effects of Dietary Phytosterols on Cholesterol Metabolism and Atherosclerosis: Clinical and Experimental Evidence." *American Journal of Medicine* 107 (1999): 588–94.

Nassr, A. O., et al. "Does Impaired Gallbladder Function Contribute to the Development of Barrett's Esophagus and Esophageal Adenocarcinoma?" *Journal of Gastrointestinal Surgery* 15 (2011): 908–14.

Nilsson, B. I., et al. "Relaltionship Between Interdigestive Gallbladder Emptying, Plasma Motilin and Migrating Motor Complex in Man." *Acta Physiology Scandinavia* 139 (1990): 55–61.

Peterson, C. T., et al. "Therapeutic Uses of Triphala in Ayurvedic Medicine." *Journal of Alternative and Complementary Medicine* 23 (2017): 607–14.

Plat, J., and R. P. Mensink. "Effects of Plant Sterols on Lipid Metabolism and Cardiovascular Risk." *Nutritional Metabolism in Cardiovascular Disease* 11 (2000): 600–601.

Plessier, J. "Comparison of the Cholecystokinetic and Choleretic Actions of Cholecystokinin, Sorbitol, Olive Oil and Magnesium Sulfate." *Pathologie Biologie* 8 (1960): 1201–10.

Portincasa, P., et al. "Impaired Gallbladder and Gastric Motility and Pathological Gastro-oesophageal Reflux in Gallstone Patients." *European Journal of Clinical Investigation* 27 (1997): 653–61.

Portincasa, P., et al. "Potential Adverse Effects of Proton Pump Inhibitors." *Current Gastroenterology Reports* 10 (2008): 208–14.

Prasad, S., and S. P. Wahi. "Pharmacognostical Investigation on Indian Sarsaparilla. 1. Root and Root-Stock of Hemidesmus indicus R." *British Indian Journal of Pharmacology* 27 (1965).

Rani, B., et al. "Triphala: A Versatile Counteractive Assortment of Ailments." *International Journal of Pharmaceutical and Chemical Sciences* 2 (2013): 101–8.

Roberts, M. S., et al. "Enterohepatic Circulation." *Clinical Pharmacokinetics* 10 (2002): 751–90.

Rose, D. P., et al. "High-Fiber Diet Reduces Serum Estrogen Concentrations in Premenopausal Women." *American Journal of Clinical Nutrition* 54 (1991): 520–25.

Samy, R. P., et al. "A Compilation of Bioactive Compounds from Ayurveda." *Bioinformation* 3 (2008): 100–10.

Schjoldager, B. T. "Role of Cholesystokinin in Gallbladder Function." *Annals of the New York Academy of Sciences* 23 (1994): 207–18.

Small, D. M., et al. "The Enterohepatic Circulation of Bile Salts." *Archives of Internal Medicine* 130 (1972): 552–73.

Thompson, J. C., et al. "Correlation between Release of Cholesystokinin and Contraction of the Gallbladder in Patients with Gallstones." *Annals of Surgery* 195 (1982): 670–76.

Tylavsky, F. A., et al. "The Importance of Calcium, Potassium, and Acid-Base Homeostasis in Bone Health and Osteoporosis Prevention." *Journal of Nutrition* 138, no. 1 (2008): 164S–65S.

Umashankar, M., and S. Shruti. "Traditional Indian Herbal Medicine Used as Antipyretic, Anticancer, Anti-diabetic and Anticancer." *International Journal of Research in Pharmacy and Chemistry* 1 (2011): 1152–59.

Whiting, K. Steven. *Controlling Cholesterol and Triglycerides*. San Diego, Calif.: Institute of Nutritional Science, 2014. https://healthyinformation.com /wp-content/uploads/2014/12/ControllingCholesterolNaturally.pdf.

Wiener, I. I., et al. "Correlation Between Gallbladder Size and Release of Cholecystokinin After Oral Magnesium Sulfate in Man." *Annals of Surgery* 197 (1983): 412–415.

Wiener, I. I., et al. "Release of Cholecystokinin in Man: Correlation of Blood Levels with Gallbladder Contraction." *Annals of Surgery* 194 (1981): 321–27.

Worning, H., and S. Mullertz. "pH and Pancreatic Enzymes in the Human Duodenum during Digestion of a Standard Meal." *Scandinavian Journal of Gastroenterology* 1 (1966): 268–83.

7. AYURVEDIC TREATMENTS FOR SPECIFIC CONDITIONS CAUSED BY THYROID DYSFUNCTION

Abascal, K., and E. Yarnell. "Nervine Herbs for Treating Anxiety." *Alternative & Complementary Therapies* 10 (2004): 309–15.

Abdell-Tawab, M., et al. "Boswellia serrata." *Clinical Pharmacokinetics* 50 (2011): 349–69.

Abraham, A. S., et al. "Magnesium in the Prevention of Lethal Arrhythmias in Acute Myocardial Infarction." *Archives of Internal Medicine* 147 (1987): 753–55.

Agarwal, S. P., et al. "Shilajit: A Review." *Phytotherapy Research* 21 (2007): 401–5.

Agnihotri, S., et al. "Chemical Composition, Antimicrobial and Topical Anti-inflammatory Activity of Jatamansi." *Journal of Essential Oil Bearing Plants* 14 (2011): 417–22.

Agular, S., and T. Borowski. "Neuropharmacological Review of the Nootropic Herb Bacopa monnieri." *Rejuvenation Research* 16 (2013): 313–26.

Ahuja, S. C., et al. "Nirgundi—Nature's Gift to Mankind." *Asian Agri-History* 19 (2015): 5–32.

Akpinar, S. "Treatment of Restless Legs Syndrome with Levodopa Plus Benserazide." *Archives of Neurology* 39 (1982): 739.

Ali, M., et al. "A Clinical Study of Nirgundi in the Management of Gridhrasi with Special Reference to Sciatica." *Ayu* 4 (2010): 456–60.

Allen, D. G., and S. Kurihara. "The Effects of Muscle Length on Intracellular

Calcium Transients in Mammalian Cardiac Muscle." *Journal of Physiology* 327 (1982): 79–94.

Allen, R. "Dopamine and Iron in the Pathophysiology of Restless Legs Syndrome." *Sleep Medicine* 5 (2004): 385–91.

Allen, R. P., and C. J. Earley. "Augmentation of the Restless Legs Syndrome with Carbidopa/Levodopa." *Sleep* 19 (1996): 205–13.

Allen, R. P., et al. "MRI Measurement of Brain Iron in Patients with Restless Legs Syndrome." *Neurology* 56 (2001): 263–65.

Ammon, H. P. T. "Modulation of the Immune System by Boswellia serrata Extracts and Boswellic Acids." *Phytomedicine* 17 (2010): 862–67.

Andersson, A. M., and N. E. Skakkebaek. "Exposure to Exogenous Estrogens in Food: Possible Impact on Human Development and Health." *European Journal of Endocrinology* 140 (1999): 477–85.

Anilakumar, K. R., et al. "Effect of Coriander Seeds on Hexachlorocyclohexane Induced Lipid Peroxidation in Rat Liver." *Nutrition Research* 21 (2001): 1455–62.

Aranha, I., et al. "Immunostimulatory Properties of the Major Protein from the Stem of the Ayurvedic Medicinal Herb, Guduchi (Tinospora cordifolia)." *Journal of Ethnopharmacology* 139 (2012): 366–72.

Aurangabad, S., et al. "Natural Memory Boosters." *Pharmacognosy Reviews* 2 (2008): 249–56.

Barnes, Mack N., et al. "Paradigms for Primary Prevention of Ovarian Carcinoma." *CA: A Cancer Journal for Clinicians* 52 (2002): 216–25.

Basch, E., et al. "Therapeutic Applications of Fenugreek." *Alternative Medicine Review* 8 (2003): 20–27.

Basler, A. J. "Pilot Study Investigating the Effects of Ayurvedic Abhyanga Massage on Subjective Stress Experience." *Journal of Alternative and Complementary Medicine* 17 (2011): 435–40.

Bernstein, L. M. "Tumor Estrogen Content and Clinico-Morphological and Endocrine Features of Endometrial Cancer." *Journal of Cancer Research and Clinical Oncology* 129 (2003): 245–49.

Beulens, J. W. J., et al. "The Role of Menaquinones (Vitamin K2) in Human Health." *British Journal of Nutrition* 110 (2013): 1357–68.

Bhalerao, S. A., et al. "Saraca asoca (Roxb), De. Wild: An Overview." *Annals of Plant Sciences* 3 (2014): 770–75.

Bharani, A., et al. "Salutary Effect of Terminalia Arjuna in Patients with Severe Refractory Heart Failure." *International Journal of Cardiology* 49 (1995): 191–99.

Biswas, K., et al. "Biological Activities and Medicinal Properties of Neem (Azadirachta indica)." *Current Science* 82 (2002): 1336–82.

Bjerver, K., et al. "Morphine Intake from Poppy Seed Food." *Journal of Pharmacy and Pharmacology* 34 (1982): 798–801.

Bolland, M. J., et al. "Calcium Supplements with or without Vitamin D and Risk of Cardiovascular Events." *British Medical Journal* 342 (2011).

Bolland, M. J., et al. "Vascular Events in Healthy Older Women Receiving Calcium Supplementation." *British Medical Journal* 336 (2008): 262–66.

Bordia, A., et al. "Effect of Ginger and Fenugreek on Blood Lipids, Blood Sugar and Platelet Aggregation in Patients with Coronary Artery Disease." *Prostaglandins, Leukotrienes, and Essential Fatty Acids* 56 (1997): 379–84.

Catanzaro, D., et al. "Boswellia serrata Preserves Intestinal Epithelial Barrier from Oxidative and Inflammatory Damage." *PloS One* 10, no. 5 (2015).

Chiang, J. P., et al. "Effects of Topical Sesame Oil on Oxidative Stress in Rats." *Alternative Therapies* 11 (2005): 40.

Chopra, R. N., et al. "The Pharmacology and Therapeutics of Boerhaavia diffusa (Punarnava)." *Indian Medical Gazette* 58 (1923): 203–8.

Christine, N., et al. "Calcium, Phosphate and the Risk of Cardiovascular Events and All-Cause Mortality in a Population with Stable Coronary Heart Disease." *Heart* 98 (2012): 926–33.

Cleland, J. G. G., et al. "Arrhythmias, Catecholamines and Electrolytes." *American Journal of Cardiology* 62 (1988): 55A–59A.

Clemens, S., et al. "Restless Legs Syndrome: Revisiting the Dopamine Hypothesis from the Spinal Cord Perspective." *Neurology* 67 (2006): 125–30.

Coskuner, Y., and E. Karababa. "Physical Properties of Coriander Seeds (Coriandrum sativum L.)." *Journal of Food Engineering* 80 (2007): 408–16.

Cundy, T., and A. Dissanayake. "Severe Hypomagnesaemia in Long-Term Users of Proton-Pump Inhibitors." *Clinical Endocrinology* 69 (2008): 338–41.

Curhan, G. C., et al. "Comparison of Dietary Calcium with Supplemental Calcium and Other Nutrients as Factors Affecting the Risk for Kidney Stones in Women." *Annals of Internal Medicine* 126 (1997): 497–504.

Curhan, G. C., et al. "A Prospective Study of Dietary Calcium and Other Nutrients and the Risk of Symptomatic Kidney Stones." *New England Journal of Medicine* 328 (1993): 833–38.

D'Angelo, E. K., et al. "Magnesium Relaxes Arterial Smooth Muscle by Decreasing Intracellular Ca2+ without Changing Intracellular Mg2+." *Journal of Clinical Investigation* 89 (1992): 1988–94.

Das, B., et al. "Clinical Evaluation of Nirgundi in the Management of Sandhivata (Osteoarthritis)." *Ancient Science of Life* 23 (2003): 22–34.

Dawson-Hughes, B., et al. "Estimates of Optimal Vitamin D Status." *Osteoporosis International* 16 (2005): 713–16.

Dean, Carolyn. *The Magnesium Miracle*. New York: Ballantine Books, 2017.

Delort, L., et al. "Central Adiposity as a Major Risk Factor of Ovarian Cancer." *Anticancer Research* 29 (2009): 5229–34.

DeLuca, H. F. "Vitamin D: The Vitamin and the Hormone." *Federation Proceedings* 33 (1974): 2211–19.

Deshmukh, S., et al. "Concept of Beauty through Ayurveda." International *Journal of Ayurveda and Pharma Research* 3, no. 9 (2015): 22–25.

De Sousa, A. "Herbal Medicines and Anxiety Disorders: An Overview." *Journal of Medicinal Plants Studies* 1 (2013): 18–23.

Dhanapakiam, P., et al. "The Cholesterol Lowering Property of Coriander Seeds (Coriandrum sativum): Mechanism of Action." *Journal of Environmental Biology* 29 (2008): 53–56.

Dhandapani, S., et al. "Hypolipidemic Effect of Cuminum cyminum L. on Alloxan-Induced Diabetic Rats." *Pharmaceutical Research* 46 (2002): 251–55.

Dhuri, K. D., et al. "Shirodhara: A Psychophysiological Profile in Healthy Volunteers." *Journal of Ayurveda and Integrative Medicine* 4 (2013): 40–44.

Divya, K., et al. "An Appraisal of the Mechanism of Action of Shirodhara." *Annals of Ayurvedic Medicine* 2 (2013): 114–17.

Dornala, S. N., and S. N. D. Snehalatha. "Multidimensional Effects of Shirodhara on Psychosomatic Axis in the Management of Psychophysiological Disorders." *International Journal of Ayurveda and Pharma Research* 2 (2014). doi:10.4172/2327-5162.S1.002

Durlach, J., et al. "Magnesium Chloride or Magnesium Sulfate." *Magnesium Research* 18 (2005): 187–92.

Earley, C. J., et al. "Abnormalities in CSF Concentrations of Ferritin and Transferrin in Restless Legs Syndrome." *Neurology* 54 (2000): 1698–700.

Ebashi, S., et al. "Calcium and Muscle Contraction." *Progress in Biophysics and Molecular Biology* 18 (1968): 123–66.

Eisner, D. A., et al. "Integrative Analysis of Calcium Cycling in Cardiac Muscle." *Circulation Research* 87 (2000): 1087–94.

Ernst, E. "Frankincense." *British Medical Journal* 337 (2008): 2813.

Ernst, E. "Herbal Remedies for Anxiety." *Phytomedicine* 13 (2006): 205–8.

Etzel, R. "Special Extract of Boswellia serrata in the Treatment of Rheumatoid Arthritis." *Phytomedicine* 3 (1996): 91–94.

Fabiato, A., and F. Fabiato. "Effects of Magnesium on Contractile Activation of Skinned Cardiac Cells." *Journal of Physiology* 249 (1975): 497–517.

Fawcett, W. J., et al. "Magnesium: Physiology and Pharmacology." *British Journal of Anaesthesia* 83 (1999): 302–20.

Firoz, M., and M. Graber. "Bioavailability of U.S. Commercial Magnesium Preparations." *Magnesium Research* 14 (2001): 257–62.

Garcia-Borreguero, D., et al. "Diagnostic Standards for Dopaminergic Augmentation of Restless Legs Syndrome: Report from a World Association of Sleep Medicine." *Sleep Medicine* 8 (2007): 520–30.

Gautam, S., et al. "Formulation and Evaluation of Herbal Hair Oil." *International Journal of Chemical Sciences* 10, no. 1 (2012): 349–53.

Gettes, L. S. "Electrolyte Abnormalities Underlying Lethal and Ventricular Arrhythmias." *Circulation* 85 (1992): 170–76.

Ghani, M. F., et al. "The Effectiveness of Magnesium Chloride in the Treatment of Ventricular Tachyarrhythmias Due to Digitalis Intoxication." *American Heart Journal* 88 (1974): 621–26.

Ghani, M. F., et al. "Effect of Magnesium Chloride on Electrical Stability of the Heart." *American Heart Journal* 94 (1977): 600–602.

Gohil, K. J., et al. "Pharmacological Review on Centella asiatica: A Potential Herbal Cure-all." *Indian Journal of Pharmaceutical Sciences* 72 (2010): 546–56.

Grases, F., et al. "Renal Lithiasis and Nutrition." *Nutrition Journal* 5 (2006): 23.

Grove, M. D., et al. "Morphine and Codeine in Poppy Seed." *Journal of Agricultural and Food Chemistry* 24 (1976): 896–97.

Guha, P. "Betel Leaf: The Neglected Green Gold of India." *Journal of Human Ecology* 19 (2006): 87–93.

Gupta, A., et al. "Indian Medicinal Plants Used in Hair Care Cosmetics." *Pharmacognosy Journal* 2 (2010): 361–64.

Gupta, A. K., and Nehal Shah. "Effect of Majja Basti and Asthi Shrinkhala in the Management of Osteoporosis." *Ayu* 33 (2012): 110–13.

Gupta, P. C. "Biological and Pharmacological Properties of Terminalia chebula Retz. (Haritaki)." *International Journal of Pharmacy and Pharmaceutical Sciences* 4, suppl. 3 (2012): 62–68.

Gupta, S. S., et al. "Effect of Gurmar and Shilajit on Body Weight of Young Rats." *Indian Journal of Physiology & Pharmacology* (1966): 87–92.

Halder, S. B., et al. "Anti-inflammatory, Immunomodulatory and Antinociceptive Activity of Terminalia arjuna Roxb Bark Powder in Mice and Rats." *Indian Journal of Experimental Biology* 47 (2009): 577–83.

Helfant, R. H. "Hypokalemia and Arrhythmias." *American Journal of Medicine* 80 (1986): 13–22.

Heymsfield, S. B., et al. "Garcinia cambogia (Hydroxycitric Acid) as a Potential Antiobesity Agent." *Journal of the American Medical Association* 280 (1998): 1596–600.

Hollifield, J. W. "Magnesium Depletion, Diuretics and Arrhythmias." *American Journal of Medicine* 82 (1987): 30–37.

Hoorn, E. J., et al. "A Case Series of Proton Pump Inhibitor-Induced Hypomagnesemia." *American Journal of Kidney Diseases* 56 (2010): 112–16.

Indurwade, N. H., and K. R. Biyani. "Evaluation of Comparative and Combined Depressive Effect of Brahmi, Shankhpushpi and Jatamansi in Mice." *Indian Journal of Medical Sciences* 54 (2000): 339–41.

Iseri, L. T., et al. "Magnesium Deficiency and Cardiac Disorders." *American Journal of Medicine* 58 (1975): 837–46.

Jadhav, V. M., et al. "Kesharaja: Hair Vitalizing Herbs." *International Journal of Pharmacological and Technical Research* 1 (2009): 454–67.

Jain, P. K., and D. Das. "The Wonder of Herbs to Treat Alopecia." *Innovare Journal of Medical Sciences* 4 (2016): 5–10.

Jain, S. B., and S. G. Chawardol. "Evaluation of Ashwagandha and Shirodhara in the Management of Depression." *International Ayurvedic Medical Journal* 2 (2014): 495–99.

Janowiak, J. J., and C. Ham. "A Practitioner's Guide to Hair Loss Part 1—History,

Biology, Genetics, Prevention, Conventional Treatments and Herbals." *Alternative & Complementary Therapies* 10 (2004): 135–43.

Jha, C. B., et al. "Bhasmas as Natural Nanorobots: The Biorelevant Metal Complex." *Journal of Traditional & Natural Medicines* 1 (2015): 2–9.

Jobling, S., et al. "A Variety of Environmentally Persistent Chemicals, Including Some Phthalate Plasticizers, Are Weakly Estrogenic." *Environmental Health Perspectives* 103 (1995): 582–87.

Joshi, A. A. "Formulation and Evaluation of Polyherbal Hair Oil." *International Journal of Green Pharmacy* 11, no. 1 (2017): S135–39.

Kadlimatti, S., et al. "Therapeutic Potentials of Ayurvedic Rasayana in the Management of Asthi Kshaya vis-a-vis Osteopenia/Osteoporosis." *Sri Lanka Journal of Indigenous Medicine* 1 (2011): 39–44.

Kapoor, R., et al. "Bacopa monnieri Modulates Antioxidant Responses in Brain and Kidney of Diabetic Rats." *Environmental Toxicology and Pharmacology* 27 (2009): 62–69.

Kar, A., et al. "Analgesic Effect of the Gum Resin of Boswellia serrata." *Life Sciences* 8 (1969): 1023–28.

Kasai, K., et al. "Forskolin Stimulation of Adenylate Cyclase in Human Thyroid Membranes." *Acta Endocrinology* 108 (1985): 200–205.

Kaushik, R., et al. "Bhasmas: The Ancient Nanopharmaceuticals." Poster. doi:10.13140/RG.2.2.34878.38726.

Kavitha, C. "Amazing Bean Mucuna pruriens." *Journal of Medicinal Plants Research* 8 (2014): 138–43.

Khosa, R. I., and S. Prasad. "Pharmacognostical Studies on Guduchi (Tinospora cordifolia)." *Journal of Indian Medicine* 6 (1971): 261–69.

Kirti, S., et al. "Tinospora cordifolia (Guduchi), a Reservoir Plant for Therapeutic Applications." *Indian Journal of Traditional Knowledge* 3 (2004): 257–70.

Krishna, K., et al. "Guduchi (Tinospora cordifolia): Biological and Medicinal Properties." *Internet Journal of Alternative Medicine* 6 (2009).

Kuanrong, L., et al. "Associations of Dietary Calcium Intake and Calcium Supplementation with Myocardial Infarction and Stroke Risk and Overall Cardiovascular Mortality in the Heidelberg Cohort of the European Prospective Investigation into Cancer and Nutrition Study." *Heart* 98 (2012): 920–25.

Kulkarni, R. R., et al. "Treatment of Osteoarthritis with an Herbomineral Formulation." *Journal of Ethnopharmacology* 33 (1991): 91–95.

Kulpers, M. T., et al. "Hypomagnesaemia Due to Use of Proton Pump Inhibitors." *Netherlands Journal of Medicine* 67 (2009): 169–72.

Kumar, P. "The Ayurvedic Bhasma: The Ancient Science of Nanomedicine." *Recent Patents on Nanomedicine* 5 (2015): 12–18.

Kumar, S. R., et al. "Shirodhara in the Management of Hypertension." *International Ayurvedic Medical Journal* 4 (2016): 79–82.

Kumar, S., et al. "In Vitro Anti-inflammatory Effects of Mahanarayan Oil

Formulations Using Dendritic Cells Based Assay." *Annals of Phytomedicine* 3 (2014): 40–45.

Kumar, V. "A Conceptual Study on Mode of Action of Nasya." *International Journal of Ayurveda and Pharma Research* 5 (2017).

Lam, Michael, and Dorine Lam. *Estrogen Dominance*. Loma Linda, Calif.: Adrenal Institute Press, 2008–2012.

Larson, C. A. "The Critical Path of Adrenocortical Insufficiency." *Nursing* 14 (1984): 66–69.

Levenson, D. I., and R. S. Bockman. "A Review of Calcium Preparations." *Nutrition Reviews* 52 (1994): 221–32.

Li, K., et al. "Associations of Dietary Calcium Intake and Calcium Supplementation with Myocardial Infarction and Stroke Risk and Overall Cardiovascular Mortality in the Heidelberg Cohort of the European Prospective Investigation into Cancer and Nutrition Study." *Heart* 98 (2012): 920–25.

Lim, T. K. "Bahinia variegate," in *Edible Medicinal and Non-Medicinal Plants*, Vol. 7, 754–65. Dordrecht, Heidelberg, London, and New York: Springer, 2014.

Lim, T. K. "Mucuna pruriens," in *Edible Medicinal and Non-Medicinal Plants*, Vol. 2, 779–97. Dordrecht, Heidelberg, London, and New York: Springer, 2012.

Litosch, I., et al. "Forskolin as an Activator of Cyclic AMP Accumulation and Lipolysis in Rat Adipocytes." *Molecular Pharmacology* 22 (1982): 109–15.

Lokhande, S., et al. "Probable Mode of Action of Nasya." *International Ayurvedic Medical Journal* 4 (2016): 359–66.

Mahboubi, M. "Rosa damascena as Holy Ancient Herb with Novel Applications." *Journal of Traditional and Complementary Medicine* 6 (2016): 10–16.

Mahmood, Z. A., et al. "Herbal Treatment for Cardiovascular Disease." *Pakistan Journal of Pharmaceutical Sciences* 23 (2010): 119–24.

Malagi, K. J., et al. "A Prospective Single Arm Open Pilot Trial to Study the Antioxidant Property of Ayurvedic Massage Therapy in Healthy Individuals." *International Journal of Pharmacology and Clinical Sciences* 2 (2013): 121–25.

Manisha, D., et al. "Role of Terminalia arjuna in Ischemic Heart Disease." *International Journal of Ayurveda and Pharmaceutical Research* 3, no. 2 (2015): 24–28.

Manjunath, A., and C. Arun. "Action of Shirodhara." *Global Journal of Research on Medicinal Plants & Indigenous Medicine* 1 (2012): 457–63.

Manson, J., et al. "Calcium Supplements: Do They Help or Harm?" *Menopause* 21 (2014): 106–8.

Maulik, S. K., et al. "Therapeutic Potential in Terminalia arjuna in Cardiovascular Disorders." *American Journal of Cardiovascular Drugs* 12 (2012): 157–63.

Meadway, C., et al. "Opiate Concentrations Following the Ingestion of Poppy Seed Products." *Forensic Science International* 96 (1998): 29–38.

Menon, M. K., and A. Kar. "Analgesic and Psychopharmacological Effects of the Gum Resin of Boswellia serrata." *Planta Medica* 19 (1971): 333–41.

Miller, G. D., et al. "The Importance of Meeting Calcium Needs with Foods." *Journal of the American College of Nutrition* 20 (2000): 168S–85S.

Mirza, A., et al. "Shilajit: An Ancient Panacea." *International Journal of Current Pharmaceutical Review and Research* 1 (2010): 2–11.

Mishra, A., et al. "Phytochemical and Pharmacological Importance of Saraca indica." *International Journal of Pharmaceutical and Chemical Sciences* 2 (2013): 1009–13.

Mishra, N. K., et al. "Anti-arthritic Activity of Boswellia serrata in Adjuvant Induced Arthritic Rats." *Journal of Pharmaceutical Education and Research* 2 (2011): 92–98.

Mizuno, S., et al. "CSF Iron, Ferritin and Transferrin Levels in Restless Legs Syndrome." *Journal of Sleep Research* 14 (2005): 43–47.

Mohapatra, H. P., and S. P. Rath. "In Vitro Studies of Bacopa monnieri—An Important Medicinal Plant with Reference to Its Biochemical Variations." *Indian Journal of Experimental Biology* 43 (2005): 373–76.

Montplaisir, J., et al. "Restless Legs Syndrome and Periodic Movements in Sleep: Physiopathology and Treatment with L-dopa." *Clinical Neuropharmacology* 9, no. 5 (1986): 456–63.

Morgan, A., and J. Stevens. "Does Bacopa monnieri Improve Memory Performance in Older Persons?" *Journal of Alternative and Complementary Medicine* 16 (2010): 753–59.

Morgan, J. P., et al. "Calcium and Cardiovascular Function: Intracellular Calcium Levels during Contraction and Relaxation of Mammalian Cardiac and Vascular Smooth Muscle as Detected with Aequorin." *American Journal of Medicine* 77 (1984): 33–46.

Murti, K., et al. "Pharmacological Properties of Boerhaavia diffusa." *International Journal of Pharmaceutical Sciences Review and Research* 5 (2010): 107–10.

Northrup, Christiane. *Women's Bodies, Women's Wisdom.* New York: Bantam Publishing, 2010.

O'Keeffe, S. T., et al. "Iron Status and Restless Legs Syndrome in the Elderly." *Age and Ageing* 23 (1994): 200–203.

Ondo, W. G., et al. "Exploring the Relationship between Parkinson's Disease and Restless Legs Syndrome." *Archives of Neurology* 59 (2002): 421–24.

Pal, D. "Bhasma: The Ancient Indian Nanomedicine." *Advances in Pharmaceutical & Technological Research* 5 (2014): 237–42.

Pal, D., and V. K. Gurjar. "Nanometals in Bhasma: Ayurvedic Medicine." *Metal Nanoparticles in Pharmacology* (2017): 389–415.

Panchabhai, T. S., et al. "Validation of Therapeutic Claims of Tinospora cordifolia." *Phytotherapy Research* 22 (2008): 425–41.

Panthi, S., and T. Gao. "Diagnosis and Management of Primary Hypothyroidism in Traditional Chinese Medicine (TCM) and Traditional Indian Medicine (Ayurveda)." *International Journal of Clinical Endocrinology & Metabolism* 1 (2015): 9–12.

Parker, W. H. "Etiology, Symptomatology, and Diagnosis of Uterine Myomas." *Fertility and Sterility* 87 (2007): 725–36.

Parkins, W. M., et al. "Comparative Study of Sodium, Chloride and Blood Pressure Changes Induced by Adrenal Insufficiency, Trauma and Intraperitoneal Administration of Glucose." *American Journal of Physiology* 112 (1935): 581–90.

Parmar, M. S. "Kidney Stones." *British Medical Journal* 328 (2004): 1420–24.

Parmley, W. W., and E. H. Sonnenblick. "Mechanisms of Contraction and Relaxation in Mammalian Cardiac Muscle." *American Journal of Physiology* 216 (1969): 1084.

Patel, J. S., and V. J. Galani. "Investigation of Noradrenaline and Serotonin Mediated Antidepressant Action of Mucuna pruriens Seeds Using Various Experimental Models." *Oriental Pharmacy and Experimental Medicine* 13 (2013): 143–48.

Patel, M. B. "Forskolin: A Successful Therapeutic Phytomolecule." *East and Central African Journal of Pharmaceutical Sciences* 13 (2010): 25–32.

Pati, D., et al. "Anti-depressant-like Activity of Mucuna pruriens, a Traditional Indian Herb in Rodent Models of Depression." *Pharmacologyonline* 1 (2010): 537–51.

Patil, V., et al. "Clinical Study on Effect of Different Methods of Shirodhara in Patients of Insomnia." *International Journal of Ayurveda and Pharma Research* 5 (2017): 28–32.

Pawar, S. D., et al. "Evaluation of Anti-inflammatory, Analgesic and Anti-arthritic Activity of Mahanarayana Oil in Laboratory Animals." *Advances in Pharmacology and Toxicology* 12 (2011): 33–42.

Pereira, J. C., et al. "Imbalance Between Thyroid Hormones and the Dopaminergic System Might Be Central to the Pathophysiology of Restless Legs Syndrome." *Clinics (Sao Paulo)* 65 (2010): 548–54.

Pike, M. C., et al. "Prevention of Cancers of the Breast, Endometrium and Ovary." *Oncogene* 23 (2004): 6379–91.

Plaza, S. M., and D. W. Lamson. "Vitamin K2 in Bone Metabolism and Osteoporosis." *Alternative Medicine Review* (2005): 24–35.

Polimeni, P. I., and E. Page. "Magnesium in Heart Muscle." *Circulation Research* 33 (1973): 367–74.

Prabhu, M. S., et al. "Effect of Orally Administered Betel Leaf (Piper betle Linn.) on Digestive Enzymes and Intestinal Mucosa and on Bile Production in Rats." *Indian Journal of Experimental Biology* 33 (1995): 752–56.

Pradhan, P., et al. "Saraca asoca (Ashoka)." *Journal of Chemical and Pharmaceutical Research* 1 (2009): 62–71.

Prakash, S. "Ashoka (Saraca indica Linn.): A Persuasive Herb for Menorrhagia." *International Journal of Applied Ayurved Research* 2, no. 2 (2015): 92–97.

Prasad, B. S., et al. "Development of a Nasya Fitness Form for Clinical Practice." *Ancient Science of Life* 34 (2014): 100–102.

Rajagopal, P. L., et al. "A Review on Nephroprotective Herbs and Herbal

Formulations." *International Journal of Pharmaceutical and Chemical Sciences* 2 (2013): 1888–904.

Ram, T. S., et al. "Pragmatic Usage of Haritaki (Terminalia chebula Retz.): An Ayurvedic Perspective vis-a-vis Current Practice." *International Journal of Ayurveda and Pharma Research* 1 (2013): 72–82.

Ramya, K. B., and S. Thaakur. "Herbs Containing L-dopa." *Ancient Science of Life* 27 (2007): 50–55.

Rana, D. G., and V. J. Galani. "Dopamine Mediated Antidepressant Effect of Mucuna pruriens Seeds in Various Experimental Models of Depression." *Ayu* 35 (2014): 90–97.

Raskar, S., and R. Shrikrishna. "Abhyanga in Newborn Baby and Neonatal Massage." *International Journal of Ayurveda and Pharma Research* 3 (2015): 5–10.

Rathi, V., et al. "Plants Used for Hair Growth Promotion." *Pharmacognosy Reviews* 2 (2008): 185–87.

Reid, I. R., and M. J. Bolland. "Calcium Supplements: Bad for the Heart?" *Heart* 98 (2012): 895–96.

Robertshawe, P. "Pharmaco-physio-psychologic Effects of Ayurvedic Oil Dripping." *Journal of the Australian Traditional Medicine Society* 15 (2009): 93.

Roden, D. M. "Magnesium Treatment of Ventricular Arrhythmias." *American Journal of Cardiology* 63 (1989): G43–46.

Roodenrys, S., et al. "Chronic Effects of Brahmi on Human Memory." *Neuropsychopharmacology* 27 (2002): 279–81.

Roy, R. K., et al. "Hair Growth Promoting Activity of Eclipta alba in Male Albino Rats." *Archives of Dermatological Research* 300 (2008): 357–64.

Saha, S., and S. Ghosh. "Tinospora cordifolia: One Plant, Many Roles." *Ancient Science of Life* 31 (2012): 151–59.

Sahu, A., et al. "Phytopharmacological Review of Boerhaavia diffusa Linn. (Punarnava)." *Pharmacognosy Reviews* 2 (2008): 14–22.

Salehi, F., et al. "Risk Factors for Ovarian Cancer." *Journal of Toxicology and Environmental Health* 11 (2008): 301–21.

Samy, R. P., et al. "A Compilation of Bioactive Compounds from Ayurveda." *Bioinformation* 3 (2008): 100–110.

Sander, O., et al. "Is Boswellia serrata a Useful Supplement to Established Drug Therapy of Chronic Polyarthritis?" *Zeitschrift fur Rheumatologie* 57 (1998): 11–16.

Saqib, M., et al. "Effect of Shilajit on Obesity in Hyperlipidemic Albino Rats." *Pakistan Journal of Medical & Health Sciences* 10 (2016): 1019–23.

Sarris, J., et al. "Plant-Based Medicines for Anxiety Disorders." *CNS Drugs* 27 (2013): 301–19.

Seamon, K. B., and J. W. Daly. "Forskolin, Cyclic AMP and Cellular Physiology." *Trends in Pharmacological Sciences* 4 (1983): 120–23.

Semwal, B. C., et al. "Alopecia Switch to Herbal Medicine." *Journal of Pharmaceutical Research & Opinion* 1 (2011).

Sengupta, K., et al. "Cellular and Molecular Mechanisms of Anti-Inflammatory Effect of a Novel Boswellia serrata Extract." *Molecular and Cellular Biochemistry* 354 (2011): 189–97.

Sethiya, N. K., et al. "An Update on Shankhpushpi, a Cognition-Boosting Ayurvedic Medicine." *Journal of Chinese Integrative Medicine* 7 (2009): 1001–22.

Sharma, K., and P. Rani. "A Holistic Ayurvedic Approach in Management of Obesity." *International Journal of Health Sciences and Research* 6 (2016): 358–65.

Sharma, L., et al. "Medicinal Plants for Skin and Hair Care." *Indian Journal of Traditional Knowledge* 2 (2003): 62–68.

Sharma, M. L., et al. "Anti-arthritic Activity of Boswellic Acids in Bovine Serum Albumin-Induced Arthritis." *International Journal of Immunopharmacology* 11 (1989): 647-52.

Sharma, M. L., et al. "Immunomodulatory Activity of Boswellic Acids from Boswellia serrata." *Phytotherapy Research* 10 (1996): 107–12.

Sharma, R. D., et al. "Effect of Fenugreek Seeds on Blood Glucose and Serum Lipids in Type 1 Diabetes." *European Journal of Clinical Nutrition* 44 (1990): 301–6.

Sharma, R. D., et al. "Hypolipidemic Effect of Fenugreek Seeds." *Phytotherapy Research* 5 (1991): 145–47.

Sharma, U. K., et al. "Role of Shirodhara with Ashwagandha in Management of Insomnia." *Environment Conservation Journal* 16 (2015): 159–63.

Shine, K. I. "Myocardial Effects of Magnesium." *American Journal of Physiology* 237 (1979): H413–23.

Siddiqui, M. Z. "Boswellia serrata, a Potential Anti-inflammatory Agent." *Indian Journal of Pharmaceutical Sciences* 73 (2011): 255–61.

Singh, C., and R. Sharma. "A Clinical Study of an Ayurvedic Formulation for the Management of Obesity." *International Ayurvedic Medical Journal* (online; 2016).

Singh, P., et al. "Lodhra: A Single Remedy for Different Ailments." *International Journal of Pharmaceutical & Biological Archives* 6 (2015): 1–7.

Singh, R. D., et al. "Seasonal Variation of Bioactive Components in Valeriana jatamansi from Himachal Pradesh, India." *Industrial Crops and Products* 32 (2010): 292–96.

Singh, S. K., and K. Rajoria. "Evaluation of Vardhamana Pippali, Kanchanar Guggulu and Kekhana Basti in the Management of Hypothyroidism." *Indian Journal of Traditional Knowledge* 14 (2015): 513–18.

Singh, S. S., et al. "Chemistry and Medicinal Properties of Tinospora cordifolia (Guduchi)." *Indian Journal of Pharmacology* 35 (2003): 83–91.

Sinha, K. K., et al. "Abhyanga: Different Contemporary Massage Technique and Its Importance in Ayurveda." *Journal of Ayurveda and Integrated Medical Sciences* 2 (2017).

Sircus, M. *Transdermal Magnesium Therapy: A New Modality for the Maintenance of Health*. Bloomington, Ind.: iUniverse Publisher, 2011.

Song, C. S., et al. "Hormones and the Liver: The Effect of Estrogens, Progestins, and Pregnancy on Hepatic Function." *American Journal of Obstetrics and Gynecology* 105 (1969): 813–47.

Soujanya, T. L., and C. H. Sadanandam. "Shirodhara—The Stress Management Therapy of Ayurveda." *International Ayurvedic Medical Journal* 5 (2017): 895–99.

Sowmya, P., and P. Rajyalakshmi. "Hypocholesterolemic Effect of Germinated Fenugreek Seeds in Human Subjects." *Plant Foods for Human Nutrition* 53 (1999): 359–65.

Subapriya, R., and S. Nagini. "Medicinal Properties of Neem Leaves." *Current Medicinal Chemistry—Anti-Cancer Agents* 5 (2005): 149–56.

Sun, E. R., et al. "Iron and the Restless Legs Syndrome." *Sleep* 21 (1998): 381–87.

Surawicz, B. "Role of Electrolytes in Etiology and Management of Cardiac Arrhythmias." *Progress in Cardiovascular Diseases* 8 (1966): 364–86.

Taghizadeh, M., et al. "Effects of the Cumin cyminum L. Intake on Weight Loss, Metabolic Profiles and Biomarkers of Oxidative Stress in Overweight Subjects." *Annals of Nutritional Metabolism* 66 (2015): 117–25.

Tandon, V. R. "Medicinal Uses and Biological Activities of Vitex negundo." *Indian Journal of Natural Products and Resources* 4 (2005): 162–65.

Tathed, P. P., et al. "Management of Systolic Hypertension with Shirodhara." *Ancient Science of Life* 32 (2012): S9.

Thakkar, J. P., and D. G. Mehta. "A Review of an Unfavorable Subset of Breast Cancer: Estrogen Receptor Positive Progesterone Receptor Negative." *Oncologist* 16, no. 3 (2011): 276–85.

Tiwle, R., and D. K. Sanghi. "Comprehensive Study of Nirgundi Plant." *Journal of Innovations in Pharmaceuticals and Biological Sciences* 2 (2015): 125–30.

Toolika, E., et al. "A Review on Ayurvedic Management of Primary Insomnia." *International Ayurvedic Medical Journal* 1 (2013): 1–5.

Turjanski, N., et al. "Striatal Dopaminergic Function in Restless Legs Syndrome." *Neurology* 52 (1999): 932.

Uebaba, K., et al. "Psychoneuroimmunologic Effects of Ayurved Oil-Dripping Treatment." *Journal of Alternative and Complementary Medicine* 14 (2008): 1189–98.

Umar, S., et al. "Boswellia serrata Attenuates Inflammatory Mediators and Oxidative Stress in Collagen Induced Arthritis." *Phytomedicine* 21 (2014): 847–56.

Upaganlawar, A., and B. Ghule. "Pharmacological Activities of Boswellia serrata Roxb." *Ethnobotanical Leaflets* 2009, no. 6, article 10 (2009).

Valette, G., et al. "Hypocholesterolemic Effect of Fenugreek Seeds in Dogs." *Atherosclerosis* 50 (1984): 105–11.

Verma, R. K., and T. Paraidathathu. "Herbal Medicines Used in the Traditional

Indian Medicinal System as a Therapeutic Treatment Option for Overweight and Obesity Management." *International Journal of Pharmacy and Pharmaceutical Sciences* 6 (2014): 40–47.

Vinjamury, S. P., et al. "Ayurvedic Therapy (Shirodhara) for Insomnia." *Global Advances in Health and Medicine* (2014): 75–80.

Wangensteen, H., et al. "Antioxidant Activity in Extracts from Coriander." *Food Chemistry* 88 (2004): 293–97.

Wilson, E., et al. "Review on Shilajit Used in Traditional Indian Medicine." *Journal of Ethnopharmacology* 136 (2011): 1–9.

Yadav, N., et al. "Development and Evaluation of Polyherbal Formulations for Hair Growth-Promoting Activity." *International Journal of Research in Applied, Natural and Social Sciences* 2 (2014): 5–12.

Zwemer, R. L. "The Adrenal Cortex and Electrolyte Metabolism." *Endocrinology* 18 (1934): 161–69.

8. DIET AND DAILY ROUTINE
FOR THYROID HEALTH

Allison, A. J., et al. "Further Research for Consideration in the A2 Milk Case." *European Journal of Clinical Nutrition* 60 (2006): 924–25.

Belury, M. A. "Dietary Conjugated Linoleic Acid in Health: Physiological Effects and Mechanisms of Action." *Annual Review of Nutrition* 22 (2002): 505–31.

Blankson, H., et al. "Conjugated Linoleic Acid Reduces Body Fat Mass in Overweight and Obese Humans." *Journal of Nutrition* 130 (2000): 2943–48.

Blasbalg, T. L., et al. "Changes in Consumption of Omega-3 and Omega-6 Fatty Acids in the United States during the 20th Century." *American Journal of Clinical Nutrition* 93 (2011): 907–8.

Blaylock, R. "Connection between MS and Aspartame." World Natural Health Organization, June 7, 2004. www.wnho.net/ms_and_aspartame.htm.

Butchko, H. H., et al. "Aspartame: Review of Safety." *Regulatory Toxicology and Pharmacology* 35 (2002): S1–93.

Byrne, Lisa Grace. *Break the Sugar Habit*. WellGroundedLife, 2017. www .wellgroundedlife.com/wp-content/uploads/2016/11/Break-the-Sugar-Habit -Workbook-2017.pdf.

Chen, C., et al. "A Mechanism by Which Dietary Trans Fats Cause Atherosclerosis." *Journal of Nutritional Biochemistry* 22 (2011): 649–55.

Chin-Dusling, J., et al. "Effect of Dietary Supplementation with Beta-casein A1 or A2 on Markers of Disease Development in Individuals at High Risk of Cardiovascular Disease." *British Journal of Nutrition* 95 (2006): 136–44.

DeLany, J. P., et al. "Conjugated Linoleic Acid Rapidly Reduces Body Fat Content in Mice without Affecting Energy Intake." *Regulatory and Integrative Physiology* 276 (1999): R1172–79.

Deth, R., et al. "Clinical Evaluation of Glutathione Concentrations after

Consumption of Milk Containing Different Subtypes of Beta-casein." *Nutrition Journal* 15 (2016): 82.

Dhaka, V., et al. "Trans Fats—Sources, Health Risks and Alternative Approach." *Journal of Food Science and Technology* 48 (2011): 534–41.

Fallon, S., and M. G. Enig. "Agave Nectar: Worse Than We Thought." *Wise Traditions in Food, Farming and the Healing Arts,* The Weston A. Price Foundation, Spring 2009.

Gupta, K., and D. S. Wagle, "Nutritional and Antinutritional Factors of Green Leafy Vegetables." *Journal of Agricultural and Food Chemistry* 36 (1988): 472–74.

Harris, W. S., et al. "Omega-6 Fatty Acids and Risk for Cardiovascular Disease." *Circulation* 119 (2009): 902–7.

Ho, S., et al. "Comparative Effects of A1 Versus A2 Beta-casein on Gastrointestinal Measures." *European Journal of Clinical Nutrition* 68 (2014): 994–1000.

Humphries, P., et al. "Direct and Indirect Cellular Effects of Aspartame on the Brain." *European Journal of Clinical Nutrition* 62 (2008): 451–62.

Jianqin, S., et al. "Erratum to: 'Effects of Milk Containing Only A2 Beta casein versus Milk Containing Both A1 and A2 Beta casein Proteins on Gastrointestinal Physiology, Symptoms of Discomfort, and Cognitive Behavior of People with Self-Reported Intolerance to Traditional Cows' Milk.'" *Nutrition Journal* 15 (2016): 45.

Joshi, K. S. "Docosahexaenoic Acid Content Is Significantly Higher in Ghrita Prepared by Traditional Ayurvedic Method." *Journal of Ayurveda and Integrative Medicine* 5 (2014): 85–88.

Kohler, J. "The Truth about Agave Syrup: Not as Healthy as You May Think." *Living and Raw Foods,* 1998. www.living-foods.com/articles/agave.html.

Laugesen, M., et al. "Ischemia Heart Disease, Type 1 Diabetes, and Cow Milk A1 Beta-casein." *New Zealand Medical Journal* 24 (2003): 116.

Lee, K. N., et al. "Conjugated Linoleic Acid and Atherosclerosis in Rabbits." *Atherosclerosis* 108 (1994): 19–25.

Leech, J. "Agave Nectar: A Sweetener That Is Even Worse Than Sugar." *HealthLine Newsletter* June 9, 2017.

Lipton, R. B., et al. "Aspartame as a Dietary Trigger of Headache." *Headache: The Journal of Head and Face Pain* 29 (1989): 90–92.

Lizhi, H., et al. "Discrimination of Olive Oil Adulterated with Vegetable Oils Using Dielectric Spectroscopy." *Journal of Food Engineering* 96 (2010): 167–71.

Maher, T. J., et al. "Possible Neurologic Effects of Aspartame, a Widely Used Food Additive." *Environmental Health Perspectives* 75 (1987): 53–57.

Majjia-Barajas, J. A., et al. "Quick Method for Determination of Fructose-Gluctose Ratio in Agave Syrup." *Journal of Food Processing and Technology* 9 (2018): 1. DOI: 10.4172/2157-7110.1000710.

McLachlan, C. N. "Beta-casein A1, Ischemic Heart Disease Mortality, and Other Illnesses." *Medical Hypothesis* 56 (2001): 262–72.

Meyer, B. J., et al. "Dietary Intakes and Food Sources of Omega-6 and Omega-3 Polyunsaturated Fatty Acids." *Lipids* 38 (2003): 391–98.

Mozafflarian, D., et al. "Consumption of Trans Fats and Estimated Effects on Coronary Heart Disease in Iran." *European Journal of Clinical Nutrition* 61 (2007): 1004–10.

Mueller, Tom. *Extra Virginity.* New York: W. W. Norton & Company, 2011.

Nicolosi, R. J., et al. "Dietary Conjugated Linoleic Acid Reduces Plasma Lipoproteins and Early Aortic Atherosclerosis in Hypercholesterolemic Hamsters." *Artery* 22 (1997): 266–77.

Noonan, S. "Oxalate Content of Foods and Effects on Humans." *Asia Pacific Journal of Clinical Nutrition* 8 (1999): 64–74.

Olney, J. W., et al. "Increasing Brain Tumor Rates: Is There a Link to Aspartame?" *Journal of Neuropathology & Experimental Neurology* 55 (1996): 1115–23.

Parodi, P. W. "Conjugated Linoleic Acid: An Anticarcinogenic Fatty Acid Present in Milk Fat." *Australian Journal of Dairy Technology* 49, no. 2 (1994): 93–97.

Remig, V., et al. "Trans Fats in America: A Review of Their Use, Consumption, Health Implications, and Regulation." *Journal of the American Dietetic Association* 110 (2010): 585–92.

Rycerz, K., et al. "Effects of Aspartame Metabolites on Astrocytes and Neurons." *NeuroPathologica* 51(2013): 10–17.

Santamaria, P., et al. "A Survey of Nitrate and Oxalate Content in Fresh Vegetables." *Journal of the Science of Food and Agriculture* 79 (1999): 1882–88.

Simopoulos, A. P. "The Importance of the Ratio of Omega-6/Omega-3 Essential Fatty Acids." *Biomedicine & Pharmacotherapy* 56 (2002): 365–79.

Soffritti, M., et al. "First Experimental Demonstration of the Multipotential Carcinogenic Effects of Aspartame Administered in the Feed to Sprague-Dawley Rats." *Environmental Health Perspectives* 114 (2006): 379–85.

Stacey, J., et al. "Health Implications of Milk Containing Beta-casein with the A2 Genetic Variant." *Critical Reviews in Food Science and Nutrition* 46 (2006): 93–100.

Sylvetsky, A. C., et al. "Understanding the Metabolic and Health Effects of Low-Calorie Sweeteners: Methodological Considerations and Implications for Future Research." *Reviews in Endocrine and Metabolic Disorders* 17 (2016): 187–94.

Tailford, K. A., et al. "A Casein Variant in Cow's Milk Is Atherogenic." *Atherosclerosis* 170 (2003): 13–19.

Taubes, G. "What if Sugar Is Worse than Just Empty Calories?" *British Medical Journal* 360 (2018).

Thom, E., et al. "Conjugated Linoleic Acid Reduces Body Fat in Healthy Exercising Humans." *Journal of International Medical Research* 29, no. 5 (2001): 392–96.

Truswell, A. S., et al. "The A2 Milk Case." *European Journal of Clinical Nutrition* 59 (2005): 623–31.

Unnevehr, L. J., et al. "Getting Rid of Trans Fats in the US Diet: Policies, Incentives and Progress." *Food Policy* 33 (2008): 497–503.

Vandana, K. S., et al. "Dinacharya Modalities to Abhyanga as a Prophylactic Measure." *International Ayurvedic Medical Journal* 5 (2017): 1–6.

Venn, B. J., et al. "A Comparison of the Effects of A1 and A2 Beta-casein Protein Variants on Blood Cholesterol Concentrations in New Zealand Adults." *Atherosclerosis* 188 (2006): 175–78.

Wertheim, Margaret L. *Breaking the Sugar Habit*. Scotts Valley, Calif.: Create Space Independent Publishing Platform, 2014.

Whitehouse, Christina R., et al. "The Potential Toxicity of Artificial Sweeteners." *AAOHN Journal* 56, no. 6 (2008): 251–59.

Wolraich, M. L., et al. "Effects of Diets High in Sucrose or Aspartame on the Behavior and Cognitive Performance of Children." *New England Journal of Medicine* 330 (1994): 301–7.

Wurtman, R. J. "Neurochemical Changes following High-Dose Aspartame with Dietary Carbohydrates." *New England Journal of Medicine* 309, no. 7 (1983): 429–30.

Zhang, X., et al. "Quantitative Detection of Adulterated Olive Oil by Raman Spectroscopy and Chemometrics." *Journal of Raman Spectroscopy* 42 (2011): 1784–88.

Index